EAT PLANTS LIFT IRON

A PLANT BASED WEIGHTLIFTING EXPERIMENT

Disclaimer: This book is not intended as a substitute for the medical advice of physicians. The reader should regularly consult a qualified physician in matters relating to his/her health and particularly with respect to any symptoms that may require diagnosis or medical attention. The information in this book is meant to inform but not advise. Like any sport, weight training poses some inherent risk. The authors and publisher advise readers to take full responsibility for their safety and know their limits. Before practicing the skills described in this book, be sure that your equipment is well maintained, and do not take risks beyond your level of experience, aptitude, training, and comfort level.

Copyright © 2015 by Boss Up Inc, Nattral Unlimited & Extreme Performance Training Systems All rights reserved. This book or any portion thereof may not be reproduced or used in any manner whatsoever without the express written permission of the publisher except for the use of brief quotations in a book review.

Library of Congress Control Number: 2014922914
Printed in the U.S.
First Printing, 2015
ISBN-10: 0983143722
ISBN-13: 978-0-9831437-2-7
Boss Up Inc
PO BOX 310330
Atlanta, Ga 31131

www.RBGFITCLUB.com
www.NATTRAL.com
www.EXTREME-FITNESS.org

Photo Credits: Larry Yanovich
Torre Washington Photo Credits: Melissa Schwartz
Layout and Design by: Mark Thomson
www.markthomson.info

 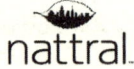 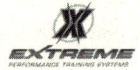 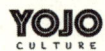

*"There's two ways to use strength;
pushing others down or lifting others up"*

- BOOKER T WASHINGTON

TABLE OF CONTENTS

	FOREWORD	I
	PREFACE	VI
	INTRODUCTION	XIX

SECTION 1: THE STUDENT IS READY

CHAPTER 1	THE SKINNY ON SOCIETY'S OBSESSION WITH SIZE	1
CHAPTER 2	TRAINING DAY	11
CHAPTER 3	BULKING/GERMAN VOLUME TRAINING	19
CHAPTER 4	MAINTAINING ON THE ROAD	41
CHAPTER 5	MAKING THE CUT (AND SHAKING THE GUT)	47
CHAPTER 6	GO HARDER	53
CHAPTER 7	LEAN BULK	59
CHAPTER 8	REACHING BIGGER GOALS	61

SECTION 2: NUTRITION GUIDELINES

CHAPTER 9	FEED THE FOCUS	65
CHAPTER 10	THE INCREDIBLE BULK PHASE	69
CHAPTER 11	NO SHORT CUTS: THE CUT PHASE MEAL PLAN	75

CHAPTER 12	GANGSTA LEAN	81
CHAPTER 13	A PROFESSIONAL WORD ON PROTEIN AND BEETS	95
CHAPTER 14	DRINK WATER	99
CHAPTER 15	REST AND RECOVERY	105
CHAPTER 16	LOOSING TO GAIN: A RECIPE FOR SUCCESS	109

SECTION 3: THE TRAINING: IRON SHARPENS MAN

CHAPTER 17	THE MAN WITH THE VEGAN IRON FISTS	135
CHAPTER 18	AIMING FOR THE GOAL	145
CHAPTER 19	THE REGIMEN	149
CHAPTER 20	FORM AND FOCUS	161
CHAPTER 21	THE BIG SIX: KEY EXERCISES FOR STRENGTH AND MASS	167
CHAPTER 22	BUILD IN BALANCE	173
CHAPTER 23	PHYSICAL CULTURE: WHY WE NEED TO GET BACK TO IT	185

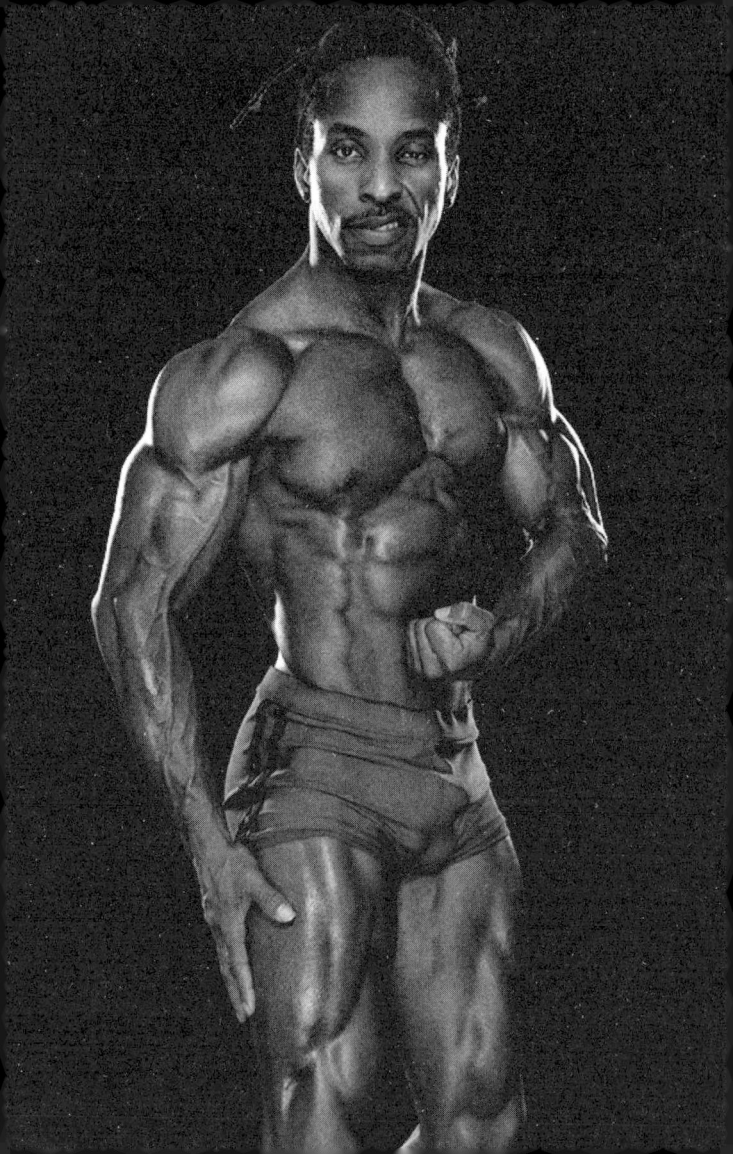

FOREWORD
BY TORRE "THA VEGAN DREAD" WASHINGTON
4 TIME PRO BODY BUILDER

Although I have been considered the top plant based competitive pro bodybuilder since 2009, written numerous articles, and was a feature and on the cover of a Special Edition of Vegan Health and Fitness magazine, this work about the future of the plant based lifestyle is truly innovative and inspiring. As an engineer by trade and a personal trainer/body sculptor by drive, I share in the enthusiasm and altruism for health and happiness for all living creatures. A success driven by passion unites our causes. Eat Plants, Lift Iron brings all the best that ties and binds us together as beings into a creative experience; a reality that makes me gracious to have met these visionaries. I am honored to be a small part of this large work of art.

> "Life is really simple,
> but we insist on making it complicated"
> – Confucius

Life starts and ends with the ground. Simple. All the nutrients that our bodies need can be found in the fruits, nuts, grains, vegetables, seeds, and legumes of the earth. The thought that we must murder another living, breathing creature to obtain nutrition (nutrition that the creature probably obtained by eating plants) is not simple...It's simple minded; as this book and the research that supports it will clarify.

Our bodies are designed to convert plants into the necessary balanced nutrition for intense training, faster recovery, and overall optimal wellness. With a balanced nutrition plan and hard work the proof will be in the (vegan) pudding.

It is well documented that developing a consistent training regimen in general will improve ones overall well-being. However, a plant-based meal plan AND a consistent training regimen can enhance all aspects of a person (physically, mentally, and spiritually).

On the physical level just to name a few, consistent weight training helps in the following ways:

- Increased bone strength and density;
- Muscle endurance; less muscle atrophy during the aging process (as compared to our non-active peers); and
- Significantly decreased risk of a plethora of preventative diseases.

Mentally the list could be as exhaustive so again let's just name a few:

- Increased oxygen and blood flow to the brain

which boosts memory and over
- All brain health;
- Improved self-esteem
- Pride in reaching a goal,
- Confidence in appearance,
- Conviction that health is the greatest wealth).

And spiritually...When you feel better and think better there is an inner peace that will guide you to more wise decisions along your journey.

The idea that a person or athlete may hear my story and be motivated; whether by curiosity, scepticism, or conviction, to see how a plant based lifestyle can not only be beneficial but also the catalyst for achieving any athletic goal they dream of is a part of my big dream come true. What makes this thing so awesome is that all of the stories of other plant based athletes and personalities have shown that a plant based lifestyle is not a hindrance but an asset. I hope we inspire others to realize that it takes only one to accomplish something before it becomes doable.

In the early to mid 1990's, HIP HOP brought us together as I blasted the motivational lyrics of Dead Prez while I crammed for exams in my college dorm room at Tuskegee University. I connected with the words of Stic and M1 on many levels. Their messages of eating to live and not living to eat was an anthem of confirmation as I began my plant based lifestyle and journey to being the best me I could be. I jumped up at the unique opportunity to attend a Dead Prez concert in which they did not disappoint. Unfortunately, that was the last time I saw them on a stage or anywhere. All I could do was just listen to their music and be inspired. Over the course of many years, my momentum and passion for lifting and plant based living lead me to as many events as possible.

I met Stic at one such event. The opportunity to meet a man who had inspired me for so many years and helped shape my life for the better stood before me in a very surreal moment. All I could think to do was ask for a picture. Thankfully Stic and his skilled, intelligent wife and nutritionist, Afya, saw past my distraction, and we were able to build a friendship based on mutual goals and passions. With a dynamic combination of my training regimen and Afya's plant based meal plans, we were able to help a new plant based athlete not only be competitive on stage but to win. Afya's knowledge and expertise of plant based nutrition was instrumental in developing that total champion package. Of course this work could not be complete without the fine tuning and personal training gifts of my fellow plant built, athlete Scott Shetler, who helped Stic (among some many others) get into the shape of his life while eating only plants.

It is with great confidence and humility that I encourage you to be open to all the knowledge these pages possess; and allow it to change your life for the better.

- Torre Washington
"Tha Vegan Dread"
4-Time Pro bodybuilder
CPT, BSME

PREFACE

"WHEN THE STUDENT IS READY THE TEACHER WILL APPEAR."

This quote is a wisdom teaching that has been around for ages and continues to prove true over and over again in my experience. I'm no believer in accidental coincidence. Things coincide because they are aligned with the Higher Purpose and Way. When I first connected with my strength coach, Scott Shetler, I knew our paths were definitely aligned. A gym owner and friend of mine named Bone breaker, who is a BIG fan of The Workout album, told me about a book project that he thought would be right up my alley. I told him it was cool to pass my info and soon after Scott reached out to me with an invite to submit an article for PLANT-BASED PERFORMANCE: A COMPASSIONATE APPROACH TO HEALTH AND FITNESS, the book he was compiling.

BOUT' THAT LIFE

As we chopped it up a bit, I learned Scott is a vegan and a successful certified personal trainer for many years with many clients of various athletic disciplines and levels. He has had extensive personal experience as a Power lifting and Kettle bell competitor and that he transitioned to an all plant based diet for ethical and health reasons. Scott told me that the profits from the book would be going to animal rights charities. His passion inspired me so I agreed to do it.

In my article I talked about the stereotypical habits of rap life that were my lifestyle at that time and how I came down with gout in my leg from the standard American diet, lack of exercise and other poor lifestyle choices. I mentioned how my wife Afya, helped me transition to a strict vegan diet to heal naturally. As a vegan I started a 10-year dedication to martial arts, over all fitness and better lifestyle choices. I gave up drinking alcohol and overtime I even stopped smoking weed. That was a toughie! Ha!

The crisis of health I experienced was actually a blessing because it shifted my path towards holistic health and wellness. I even became an avid distance runner and trained myself to complete a full 26.2-mile marathon nonstop. As I was thinking back working on my article for Scott's book on plant based performance, and reflecting on the many positive changes I had made in my lifestyle, there was one change that came to mind that I had yet to fulfil. And so I had an idea for an experiment.

VISION FOR GROWTH

Even through all my training, my physical frame was still not where I desired it to be. I still felt underweight and too skinny. It was not so much that I was comparing myself to others but just for my own personal goals and how I see myself, I wanted to make some changes. I had never dedicated myself to really trying to bulk up with a serious commitment. Lifting iron just didn't hold my interest for more than a spontaneous session here or there. I had been totally immersed into fitness through martial arts, running, yoga and calisthenics for years, but weight lifting was never something that I had embraced consistently. And though I felt like I was truly in the best shape of my life as a long distance runner, I new I had plenty of room to develop more muscle. In fact, that's an understatement.

A CUSTOM APPROACH

I didn't just want to add on muscle any old kind of way. I've learned to approach my health holistically. So if I was going to attempt to gain some weight, I was thinking that 20lbs would be significant enough; I'd have to do it on holistically healthy terms. I didn't just want a cosmetic difference; I wanted a qualitative difference without sacrificing my values of well-rounded, well-being. So the hypothesis for my experiment began unfolding.

CAN'T STOP RUNNING

I took into consideration that my metabolism has always been very high, and to add to that my long distance running burns tons more calories. So the obvious thing to do would be to cut out all of the running to make gaining weight easier, right? No, thanks! Not going to happen. No, sir. My approach to training is about being sustainable as a long-term lifestyle for me. Running is an integral part of my life that I value and didn't feel was negotiable. So I decided I'd have to do it in a way that I wouldn't have to give up my running. I needed a strategy that integrated well with how I live and what my values are. And so, as my list of stipulations grew so did the difficulty of the challenge.

NO SYNTHETIC SUPPLEMENTS

Another stipulation was that I knew I didn't want to take any supplements or any of those synthetic powders. In fact, I didn't even want to use the organic ones or even the organic plant based powders of any kind. I wanted my experiment to be with just real whole food. Let me explain why.

My family physician is Dr. Wu, an acupuncturist and herbalist who practices Eastern medicine. She put me up on game from the Traditional Chinese Medicine perspective awhile back about how the powders and supplements and even vitamins overwork the kidneys and the liver processing all those high dosages of chemical concoctions made in a lab or factory and that they can cause all kinds of imbalances in the internal system. She taught me about how the body is designed to extract the amount of nutrients it needs from whole foods in a way that does not over tax the organs. She explained that the scientists of the Western Medicine paradigm have come up with these synthetics and powders to "sneak pass" the bodies natural regulation system, to get right into the bloodstream. This becomes toxic over time. She said that they sell this stuff because it appeals to the western imbalanced notion of "more is better for you" but that's not always the case. Dr. Wu taught me that much of Western medicine has plenty of intelligence but often runs low on wisdom.

TO EACH THEIR OWN

Now before I am accused of heresy, by my friends out there who are die-hard plant protein supplement takers let me say this. There are those who have serious illnesses who have benefited from the boosts from whole food organic plant based supplementation. There are those of the opinion that we need to take extra vitamins and powders etc. to supplement and avoid deficiencies because there is less quality of nutrients in the soil and therefore less absorption of nutrients by the body from modern whole foods, especially as vegans. I'm certainly no authority on the issue and I'm open to all sides and recognize there are many layers to an onion. I'm not anti-supplements if they are whole food plant based and organic and taken in moderation or to support healing of serious illnesses.

SUPER FOODS

A much better and more holistic option than these synthetic, extracted, highly processed, isolated chemical concoctions are natural whole food organic "super foods" such as chia, flax and hemp seeds or maca root or goji berries and so on. These may be ground up into powdered forms for smoothies and shakes but they still have all the whole food content in tact and are not isolated and processed chemically like synthetic supplements are. What I know for sure is that if I can get my nutrition and energy from a real whole food, I'm banking on that because that's what my body was naturally designed for. I'm going to trust Nature's intelligence. I'm clear that profit motives have been known to interfere with and even be the culprit behind certain scientific "findings". But, hey to each his own. I don't want to convince anyone to stop taking supplements if that's your choice, but I do want to be clear on why I chose to avoid them for this experiment. I am excited to share the positive results achieved in spite of not using them.

VEGAN: WHAT'S FISH GOT TO DO WITH IT?

Thanks to my wife's professional nutritional guidance and support, my diet has remained balanced and healthy over the years. But at some point I started developing eczema like allergies for wheat gluten and then all nuts except peanuts. When I cut those allergens out of my diet, my allergic symptoms went away. But with out the seitan and other wheat gluten based veggie "meat" products and no almonds, or almond milk or almond butter which I loved, I would have fewer options as a vegan and be getting a lot less protein in my diet.

As I stated already I didn't want to go hard on protein supplements and I wanted more variety than just tofu and beans, so, with the consent of my vegan nutritionist, and physician, I re-incorporated wild caught fish into my diet.

Pesca-Vegan is what I call this fish and plant based hybrid diet because it was still no dairy, cheese ever, all plant based and animal free otherwise, but I respect the fact that Vegans for ethical reasons would feel that it is an oxymoron to call yourself a vegan if you eat fish. I don't mean to claim to be something that I'm not at all, nor to offend those dedicated to the Vegan cause for ethical reasons. I use the term because how I learned to distinguish vegan from vegetarian was that vegans don eat eggs or dairy, and so in that way I use it. Again, not looking to form a Pesca Vegan cult, lol, I'm just clarifying my use of the term because having been a strict vegan, for health reasons for 10 years I met many Vegans who educated me on the ethical motivations behind many who embrace the vegan lifestyle.

100% VEGAN

I reached out to Scott, and I told him that I wanted to gain some weight and learn the Iron Culture. I told him I was eating my self described pesca vegan diet and that I was gluten free and allergic to tree nuts, I didn't want to take supplements or powders of any kind and that as a distance runner I wanted to maintain my long distance endurance conditioning. Scott seemed to be un-phased by my host of stipulations. He suggested but didn't insist that it would be cool to see what would be the outcome if I'd stop eating fish and go back to 100% vegan. And I agreed.

So we decided I'd go 100% vegan, no fish, supplements, powders, gluten or nuts (except peanuts). He said he wasn't a nutritionist but could give me general dietary pointers from a plant-based perspective and I said I think I have the perfect person to help us in that arena, my wife Afya.

WIFE AND NUTRITIONIST: BEST OF BOTH WORLDS

I asked Afya to join us on our experiment as my nutritionist. She has always been that for me anyway since we first met long before she got her Bachelor's Degree in Nutrition and Holistic Health Counsellor certification and became a wellness professional, chef and author. She was a vegetarian when we met back in the ancient times of the early 90's and she has been teaching me through example and encouragement about the healthy lifestyle from our first date and ever since.

Afya and I have been together over two decades and I've witnessed and supported her following her calling for nutritional excellence. I saw her put in the grind time day and night going to school and get certified as a holistic Health Counsellor in New York at the Institute of Integrative Nutrition. I was there seeing her supremely dedicated work ethic as she got her degree in Nutrition from Georgia State University.

From cookbooks to counselling to educational workshops, Afya has been an inspiration to me and many others and she makes it so simple and practical and fresh the way she shares and presents her wisdom. She has healed, educated, and empowered so many of our loved ones as well as clients from fitness models, to pregnant mothers, to WIC recipients, to celebrity artists including myself.

I knew she'd get a kick out of all the calculations and scientific details of the experiment because she's into all of that kinky nerdy scientific stuff. So when I asked her she accepted but with one stipulation: only if I do what she tells me. How could I not agree when I'm getting a nutritionist, personal chef and sexy love goddess all in one? Hmmmm. OK, you drive a hard bargain but it's a deal.

I'm so blessed to have a woman in my life with so much talent and intelligence that nourishes and supports me and helps keep me on my "A-game". I'm OK with sharing the nutritional science and cooking tips that she developed for this experiment, but you'll have to find you a sexy love goddess somewhere else! Lol!

So, boom! Three the hard way! I got my dream team together and Scott projected we would shoot to reach our goal of twenty pounds in about 4 months. No turning back. Time to get my mind right and get ready for this Iron.

XVII

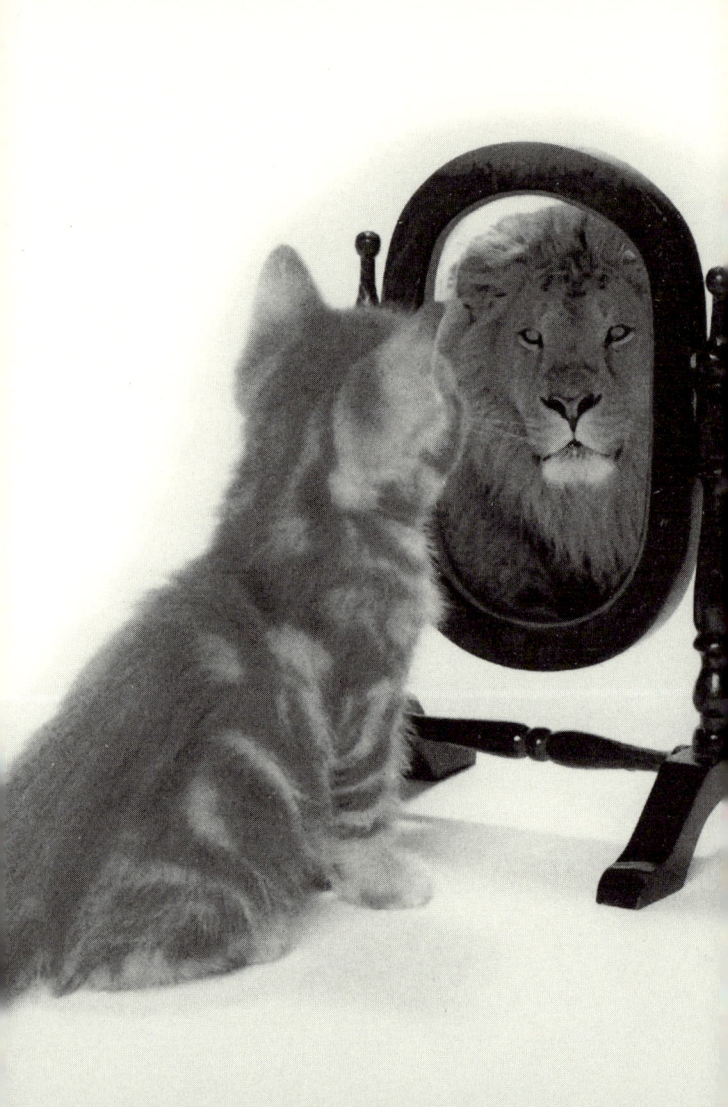

INTRODUCTION

LION HEART

Have you ever seen the picture of the domesticated house cat that catches a glimpse of himself in the mirror? He doesn't see a domesticated house cat, when he looks at his image in the mirror, he sees a Lion. I've always been inspired by that photo because it reminds me of what my Mom told me over and over growing up. "It's not how others see you, it's how you see yourself."

ACTIONS SPEAK LOUDEST

Nobody needs to convince you that you have the spark of possibility to reach and realize greater and greater levels of your potential. Deep inside you know it instinctively and you know you are supposed to discover it! What I do want to emphasize is the turning of that spark of possibility into a burning flame of action.

NO HOCUS POCUS

Taking action is what makes our potential manifest. Taking action is how what's possible, become actuality. Taking action is what makes the difference between having whatever our highest desires in life are as opposed to just thinking about it and wishing, wanting and waiting on it to magically happen. The real magic wand is the sincerity of the desire in your heart. The magic happens when the action happens. When that burning passion in the heart ignites and fuels action nothing can stop you. When we firmly make up the mind to act on what we desire to manifest, we are unstoppable. In fact, as the great author Paulo Coelho so eloquently put it "the Universe will conspire to help you." Of course, we will meet challenges as it goes in all worthwhile journeys and adventures. The task is to allow the challenges to strengthen us. Eat Plants, Lift Iron is a walk down that epic road of Transformation.

MORE THAN A MUSCLE PLAN

If you think this book is going to be about a quick and easy new way to gain some muscle, you are in for a surprise. You are about to experience an inner journey with me. You are going to see the path I took, step by step, from my personal perspective as well as the professional perspective of the experts on my team. But the real takeaway is about you seeing how this all relates and resonates to your life. The main reason we all took the time and made the effort to bring this book about is to provide you with insights, experience and expertise. I've gotten so many requests for this kind of in-depth information and we hope that it can serve your needs well.

I'M NOT A BODYBUILDER

I'm not a bodybuilder or power lifter. I have humongous respect for the discipline these guys and girls have for such a demanding lifestyle. What I have done with this experiment is not to say I have become a power lifter or bodybuilder, because I surely haven't. That's a whole other level that while I admire the lifestyle tremendously, I don't feel it is necessary for health or fitness or building more muscle. Those are great sports when done with a sense of inner balance and great ways to develop and maintain incredible strength and amazing physiques!

My experiment is much more scaled down. I'm a runner who wanted to see if I could add on about 20 pounds and see some muscle on my body for a change, on a gluten free, tree nut free, vegan diet. My restrictions and stipulations and lifestyle may not be identical to yours or what you want to accomplish. That's fine. I simply offer something I think everyday skinny guys can relate to and see that even with all those "stipulations" I had, that gains are achievable without taking drugs or gorging out on animal products or synthetic powders or pills. You don't have to sacrifice the quality of your health to build quality of muscle.

The greatest of our strength comes from within. The inner strength is that inner self-confidence to love ourselves as we are and be happy and grateful for that, skinny or not.

It's not about having an unhealthy obsession to become some perfect image of external physique. When the goals we aspire to achieve can provide us a means by which to develop ourselves from the inside out, in a healthy way I think that is a takeaway that applies in life universally.

Scott, Afya and myself are sharing real life experience as just a small example of what can be done when you make up the mind to get it done. This is not a book about bodybuilding. But it does involve building the body. This is not a book about power lifting but it does involve empowering and uplifting oneself to reach greater potential. Training with Scott has helped me to see so many parallels and metaphors that the Iron reveals for Life. My intention is that this book can inspire you to have greater acceptance and faith in yourself and give you some tools to build and sculpt and reveal the empowered YOU, that you know is in there.

THE DRAGON GUARDS THE GOLD

In this journey you will walk beside me as I face the adventure, beasts, demons and challenges on the way to my destination. You will see how passage through one door to the next is hard earned and not given and every arrival is just a beginning of yet another journey.

You are familiar with epic voyages for treasure, and this is surely one of those epic journeys. Remember that the Dragon guards the gold. To get to the gold, or should I say goal, the Dragon that stands in the way, must be slayed. So get ready for Beast Mode.

HOW THIS BOOK IS SET UP

This book is set up in 3 main sections for your convenience. We wanted to make it practical for you to reference the information.

THREE SECTIONS:

(STIC) THE STUDENT IS READY

The first section is my narrative of what I went through, how I maintained my motivation, how I adapted to the training and the results I experience physically and beyond.

(AFYA) NUTRITION GUIDELINES

The Second section is Afya's perspective on the Nutritional game plan she developed and how it worked and was adjusted to accommodate my changing needs. She provides lots of nutritional tips and pointers as well.

(SCOTT) IRON SHARPENS MAN

The third section, Scott lays out the nitty gritty of the actual training regimen that he designed for me, the scientific rationale behind it, and the results that we achieved through each phase. Scott also shares a gang of practical tips and valuable insights for Iron training in general.

At the conclusion of each section, we sum up with some key takeaways.

With gratitude, humility and profound reverence for the Iron and all those who work with it to build their minds, muscles and motivate others, I welcome you to experience our experiment EAT PLANTS, LIFT IRON.

Khnum "stic" Ibomu
Hip Hop Artist, Founder of RBG FIT CLUB

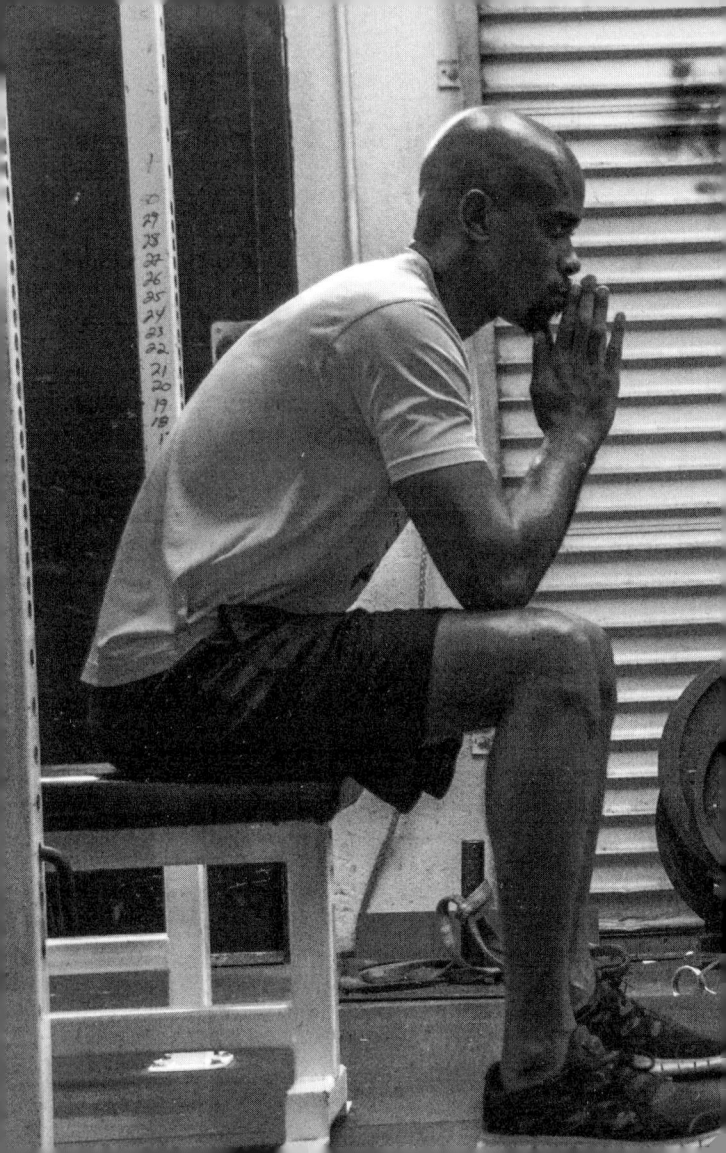

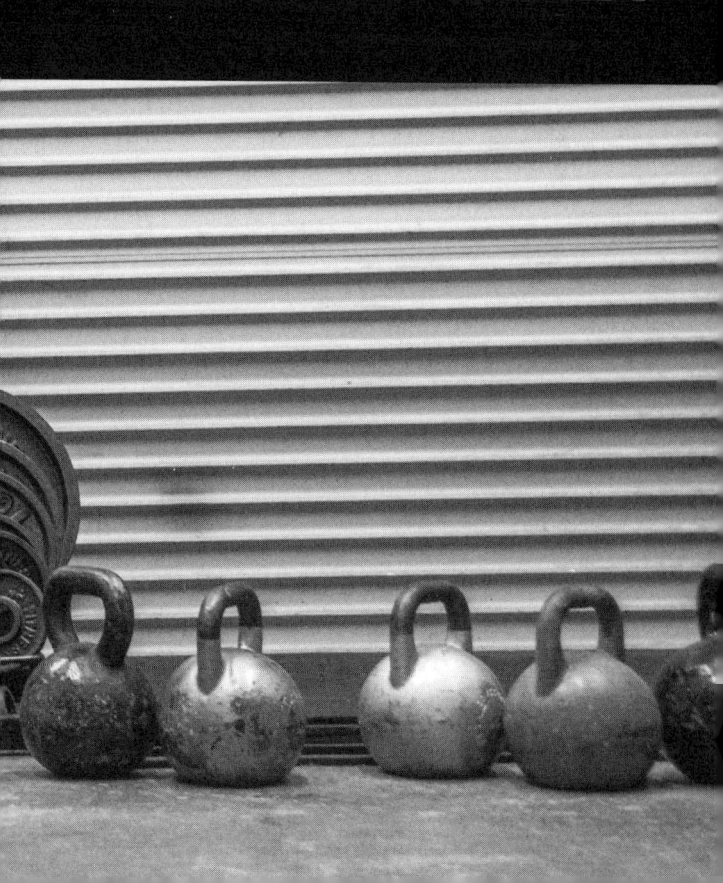

SECTION 1: STIC OF DEAD PREZ
THE STUDENT IS READY

THE STUDENT IS READY

CHAPTER 1
THE SKINNY ON SOCIETY'S OBSESSION WITH SIZE

I had to be no older than seven or eight, flipping through the pages of my comic books while visiting at my Grand Mama's house. She was looking through one of her Finger Hut catalogs and I was zoned out in my comic book world. I came across this cartoon advertisement where this skinny kid is hanging out at the beach and this muscle bound dude comes along and kicks sand in his face and all the pretty girls in bikinis start laughing. The skinny kid goes off and orders this book for 25 cents that promises to teach him how to get some big ass muscles like Charles Atlas. Well not in those words but that's how my mind remembers it!

The skinny kid follows the scrawny to brawny program and in what seemed like an instant this once puny little kid who had been ridiculed with sand kicked in his face and played in front of these chicks, now has muscles popping out of his ass every where. He goes back to the beach, punks the meathead who had intimidated him before and now the chicks were digging him!

"Grandma! Can I have 25 cents"?
"For what, baby?"

THE STUDENT IS READY

"I want to get muscles!"
I showed her the advertisement and she agreed to give me the quarter, helped me fill out the form and gave me an envelope and a stamp. I put that quarter in the envelope like I was stranded on an island sending out a distress signal! I raced it to her mailbox and pushed the red flag up so the mailman would know this is some important shit and to hurry up and come get it!

I was so excited to transform my skinny body into what I had seen in that cartoon ad!
Every few days I'd ask my grandma did my book come yet.
"No baby not yet."

Week later, I'd be over visiting.
"Did it arrive Grand ma?"
"Not yet baby."
Weeks later. I'd call her on the telephone.
"I'm sure you got it by now right grandma?"
"No baby I haven't seen it."

Months go by. No package in the mail for me. I finally realized it was never going to arrive.

I had got my hopes up waiting on that book to come. It was a promise that I would become something more. I felt like Charles Atlas not only stole my quarter but also my dream.

NOT SO SUPER SELF IMAGE

My family nickname was Peewee and I always secretly hated that. That ain't no name that you want to be called as a young dude. But I guess it was fitting. As a really thin kid, I felt my head looked too big for my body and my clothes would always fit funny cause my limbs were long but my waist and torso was so thin. It was a challenge to find clothing that complimented my frail frame. I used to just tell my Mom get whatever she likes for school shopping. I didn't even care. My feet were big as my older brother's feet and he's eight years old than me! I just felt awkward and lanky. With the promise of Charles Atlas' book, I thought I found a way I could be more like the superheroes in my comic books. I was going to be liked and admired. I was going to be super. I was going to stop being called Peewee! I was going to surprise everyone. I was going to be special. But the book never arrived. I was so let down. Still the same old skinny kid I ever was, as Charles Atlas put it, just a scrawny old weakling, who girls laugh at and big muscular guys make fun of. I didn't tell my grandma this of course but with all my little 8-year-old heart all I could muster up to think was fuck Charles Atlas! Seriously though, years later as I would visit my grandma, I'd often think about what would've happened had my book came.

THE STUDENT IS READY

SKINNY BOYS

As I've continued to live life, I discovered that I had become identified and attached to what I call a "skinny agreement" or "a skinny guy's complex". My self-image as being "too slim" or "too thin" was shaped by the social beliefs I was raised in, as well as my own ego buying into it and feeding it. My feelings and judgments about a thin physical frame, and the social feedback I got about it, corresponded in a way that has affected my self-esteem for many years.

I'd wear layers of over sized clothing to make my self appear less frail. I'd have on 4x sized T-shirts when I actually could fit a small. I'd wear size 38 pants when my actual waist size was probably 10 sizes smaller. But I didn't want to wear anything that revealed the actual size of my thin body.

I used to say to myself in my early teens when I'm older I wonder will I EVER look like a muscular adult male. I saw my older brother lifting weights and getting nice results in his upper body size and definition. He'd be out in the yard with free weights. He used two cinder blocks and wooden board for a bench. He was always putting in work with some of our cousins and other friends from the neighborhood. I was intimidated to even try to workout with him. I thought I would embarrass myself with not even being able to lift the least amount of weight.

My cousin Lomax was around my brother's age and he was what we called hood swole. We all thought his physique was the closest thing we'd ever seen to Lou Ferrigno, the actor who played the original Incredible Hulk on the television series. I would listen how the girls would swoon and speak so fondly about Lomax muscular body and the more they praised him, the more my fragile ego judged my body as the opposite.

My cousins would also tease me a lot. I remember having my shirt off on one of those hot Florida summer days and being at my Aunts' house hanging out with my cousins. I was the joke of the moment when one of my cousins said you are the winner of the Mr.Puny-Verse contest. Not Mr. Universe, puny-verse! I learned to believe that in the category of musculature, I was a loser.

I concluded from the comic books I read and the TV shows we watched and the messages we were bombarded with, that masculinity means big ass muscles! I erroneously inferred that muscle equals Manhood. So to be a growing boy and to be thinner than Olive Oil from the Popeye's cartoon definitely didn't enhance my self-esteem at all.

ROLE OF ADVERTISING IN SELF-IMAGE.

In revisiting some of those psychological issues I had as youth, which I sensed may be widely common,

THE STUDENT IS READY

I did some further research and interestingly enough that little old Charles Atlas advertisement is one of the most successful mail order campaigns ever created. Millions and millions of his books were sold to skinny little guys like me who wanted a way out of the shame and insecurity that his psychological cartoon so shrewdly capitalized on.

Countless famous athletes have confessed to being adherents to Mr. Atlas' "dynamic tension" approach to physical training. It's not that I think that it wasn't a good thing to offer a physical development program. I just want to point out the psychological aspects it exploited in making it such a success.

The marketing approach was aimed at young boys and so comic books full of big brawny superheroes were the best place to have a captive, instantly receptive audience. The scenario on the beach, made the young person see themselves in an emotionally vulnerable way and then boom, "Grandma, I need 25 cents!" It's not like it was promoted like "for your health try this program" it was aimed at the fragile ego of the skinny guy, reinforcing the stereotype of no muscles equals no manhood. I learned that there was actually a lot of research done on this psychological issue and it has a name; Muscle Dysmorphia.

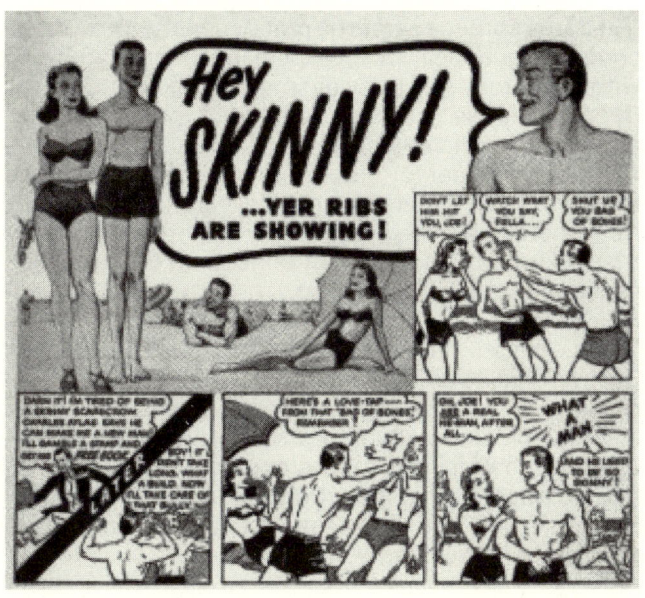

MUSCLE DYSMORPHIA

Muscle Dysmorphia, sometimes referred to as the Adonis Complex, is a psychological disorder in which a person becomes obsessed with the idea that they are not muscular enough.

THE STUDENT IS READY

"In this disorder a person is preoccupied with thoughts concerning appearance, especially musculature. As with other forms of body dysmorphic disorder, Muscle Dysmorphia is strictly connected with selective attention: individuals selectively focus their attention on perceived defect (too skinny body, underweight etc.). They are hyper-vigilant to even small deviations from perceived ideal and they ignore information that their body image is not consistent with reality." – Anthony Cortese, Sociologist.

Sociologists like Anthony Cortese view Muscle Dysmorphia as an obsessive-compulsive disorder that reflects the dysfunction of gender roles in modern society. Muscular Dysmorphia is primarily a male disorder that is the mirror opposite of a primarily female anorexia nervosa, Cortese says. "These men are obsessed with attaining an unrealistic cultural standard of muscularity as masculinity."

Several factors influence the development of Muscle Dysmorphia including: Culture, Biological predisposition, Psychological vulnerabilities (e.g. Low self-esteem) and early traumatic childhood experiences (e.g. Bullying and teasing).

Other findings went on to say that Muscle Dysmorphia can manifest as an exaggerated emphasis on appearance, physical strength and attractiveness. For instance, people compare themselves with idealized cultural figures such as unattainably muscular heroes in children's books, comics and action figures. Muscle Dysmorphia influences a person's mood, often causing depression or feelings of disgust. Individuals repeat negative and distorted self-statements concerning their appearance to such an extent that they become automatic. This is often connected with constant comparing of a person's body to an unattainable ideal.

Perhaps you can relate to some degree or another in your own self-image and experiences. As I trained during this experiment, I've had to dig deep into my own psyche, stir up and that contributed heavily to shaping my early self-image.

SELF-AWARENESS; SELF-ACCEPTANCE

The takeaway I want to give you is this. There are people pushing all kinds of programs to exploit our psychological vulnerabilities to sell us whatever they are selling but for a well-rounded well-being approach to training it's important to have our own affirming motivations. It's important that we train with a sense of enjoyment and appreciation and not an obsessive urgency because we are unhappy with ourselves.

There is nothing wrong with gaining muscle, training hard and reaching goals. But I want to be clear that it's not the muscles or how much we weigh or don't weigh or any other aspect of physical appearance that

THE STUDENT IS READY

makes us valuable or worthy and powerful. We are valuable, worthy and powerful innately. How we see ourselves psychologically and spiritually empowers us and if we choose to grow and shape our muscles then that is a reflection of our inner values and not the other way around.

It's essential to have a healthy self image that is based on accepting who you are as you are. As I said in my song Back on my Regimen "Strength comes from within, it's not the outer image."

Let's enjoy, work hard, and push to reach our goals but be mindful that value is not something we should seek from the results of our training or our physical appearance at all. We are already valuable and powerful. It is through expanding the size of our values of character not just the size of our muscles, that we manifest our highest potential. But make no mistake me and Charles Atlas got some unfinished business. Let's go!

CHAPTER 2
TRAINING DAY

"The purpose of training is to tighten up the slack, toughen the body, and polish the spirit."
- MORIHEI UESHIBA

Scott and I agreed that 9 am would be the best time for my weekly sessions on Monday, Wednesday and Fridays. But Scott's gym Extreme Performance Training Systems is an hour away from my house. Since I take my son to school on those mornings as well and morning traffic is like watching a colony of snails migrate uphill, my day would have to start by 6 am. That was the only way I would have enough time to get my son up, fed and dropped to school and then get to Scott's in the snail paced morning rush by 9 am.

This also meant I would have to significantly alter my night owl style of working and be in bed by 10:30pm to get 7-8 hours of optimal sleep. That was a BIG switch for me because as a songwriter and producer and an avid nighttime reader, my creative juices and curiosities would just start flowing at midnight or thereafter.

So the first challenge that I got even before touching a weight. I had to prioritize my time around the gym and create new sleeping habits to accommodate my goal.

THE STUDENT IS READY

> **IF YOU HAVE A GOAL TO ACHIEVE SOMETHING, YOU MUST BE WILLING TO ADJUST AND ADAPT TO WHATEVER HAS TO HAPPEN TO MAKE IT HAPPEN.**

PREPPING THE NIGHT BEFORE

To save time, on the evening before my training days I'd layout my gym clothes and throw some big yams in the oven and by the time the yams were done, id be showered up and meditated and ready to shut it down for the night. By having the yams already prepared the night before, heating them up for breakfast only took minutes. This gave me time to meditate, make my big smoothie and my son's breakfast and pack his lunch and get all of the other morning essentials done and out the front door on time.

MORNING COMMUTE

Initially, during the bulking phase which I will go into more detail about in a bit, my most typical breakfast regimen would be a big smoothie with blueberries, banana, peanut butter, pumpkin seeds, hemp seeds, fresh ginger and other fruit depending on what was in the freezer. Then I'd eat two to three huge baked yams covered with raw pumpkins seeds, cinnamon and maple syrup. I'd also have 20oz or so of water and a big thermos full of hot yerba mate herbal tea and hemp milk. I'd mix it up here and there but that was my most basic simple and easy go to meal, for that early in the am. Over time I learned that the yams gave me the perfect amount of fuel to feel strong and energized under the iron. If I didn't have my yams I could tell the difference. I'd pack whatever I didn't finish from my morning meal by out the door time in a recycled to go container and me and my son would jump in the jeep and get the day cracking.

I enjoyed the morning drive to drop my son off to school. We'd crack jokes and eat whatever was unfinished of our breakfasts on our laps, listening to music or audio books or just being present in silence.

We'd pull up to his charter school campus, with other middle schoolers swarming around and see other parents in long lines of cars making their drop offs. I'd give him a pound, we'd say I love you, and I'd watch him go into his homeroom. Then I get in focus mode for the school of Iron.

LIBRARY ON WHEELS

Traffic early in the morning is a long slow stop and go creeping all the way up highway 285 but I made use of the time by feeding myself positive content. Since I had an hour commute, I pre-planned my "mental breakfast" by having audio books, TED Talks and other motivational YouTube videos book-marked so I could

THE STUDENT IS READY

listen to the audio on the drive. I keep an ongoing collection of affirming selections and schedule them in when I have things to do like travel or wait in a line etc. My appetite for practical knowledge is even more voracious than my appetite for food. The auxiliary port in my Jeep Wrangler connects to my phone so I have a vast library at a touch away.

Song ideas would also be flowing and so I would jot down ideas and lyrics as I sat in these long stops. It became my morning ritual sipping tea from my stainless steel Stanley thermos. By the time I would get to the gym an hour away, I was inspired, nourished, energized and ready to move from all that sitting!

FIRST IMPRESSIONS

The first day I arrived at Extreme Performance Training Systems, it took me a bit to find it. I missed my turn several times and had a challenge getting back to the access road off the freeway. I phoned Scott and he patiently guided me back on the right path and I finally pulled up in front of the gym. Extreme Performance Training Systems is in an office park next to a small car dealership run by some African brothers. You wouldn't think that there was a gym in this complex, but believe me when I tell you, it goes down.

STIC'S BIG ASS YAMS AND PUMPKIN SEEDS RECIPE

2-3 Big ass yams
½ Cup Raw pumpkin seeds
Pinch of Cinnamon per Yam
1 Tsp Earth Balance Non dairy spread per yam
Maple Syrup to taste

1. Preheat oven to 450
2. Wash yams to remove dirt
3. Bake for 45-50 minutes
4. Remove Yams on to a plate
5. Slice yams open and add Earth Balance Non dairy spread, maple syrup
6. Sprinkle Pumpkin seeds evenly distributed on Yams

Nutrients per serving:
Calories 585
Fat 22g
Carbs 80g
Protein 21

THE STUDENT IS READY

EXTREME PERFORMANCE TRAINING SYSTEMS

I opened the glass door and walked into to the brightly lit carpeted front room where there is various fitness equipment, machines, dumbbell racks, balance balls, kettle bells, heavy bags, books, an office computer center and a red punching dummy that looked like he is used to getting punched in the face. There is also a lot of Spider man memorabilia.

Scott has two full sleeves of tattoos, baldhead and clean-shaven, and has this rock and roll edged, Shaolin Monk coolness about him. Good vibes right off the bat. He gives me a tour of the facility.

There is a nice glass paned refrigerator next to a wooden door leading to an industrial looking warehouse space, about 500 x 500 feet that has a huge garage type retractable door. In the warehouse area, there is cement flooring, a couple squat cages, multiple flooring mats, pull up stands with Lifeline USA's Jungle Gym suspension straps hanging from them, more kettle bells, dead lift bars and other gym equipment.

There is a chalkboard with the Chinese character for strength drawn in chalk on it as well as current lifting stats and gym records. On the surrounding walls are various motivational posters of legendary power lifters, more Spider man collectibles and Henry Rollins and The Rollins Band vintage touring posters. I learned Scott used to be a drummer in a hard-core punk band and is a huge fan of all types of music.

FIRST THINGS FIRST

Since it was my first day, Scott said that he wanted to start off with taking my body measurements and he started a Google document to keep a record of our progress. He measured my weight on a digital scale and then took measurements of my body mass index by pinching my stomach, inner thigh and chest with this contraption called a calliper, I think, that looked like an extra strength salad tong. He said the first weeks or so was going to be kind of an assessment period where he could see where I was currently at strength and energy wise, calculate my current strength levels and tweak my plan more accurately once he collected certain preliminary data from my performance.

The training the first week or so was nothing too intense. I learned basic form and breathing techniques and I went through a moderate amount of sets of core exercises such as squat, bench, and dead lifts. I felt slightly sore but nothing too significant. I went on my regular long distance runs on days in between the weight training. I did this basic routine for about two or three weeks just kind of acclimating my body to the iron.

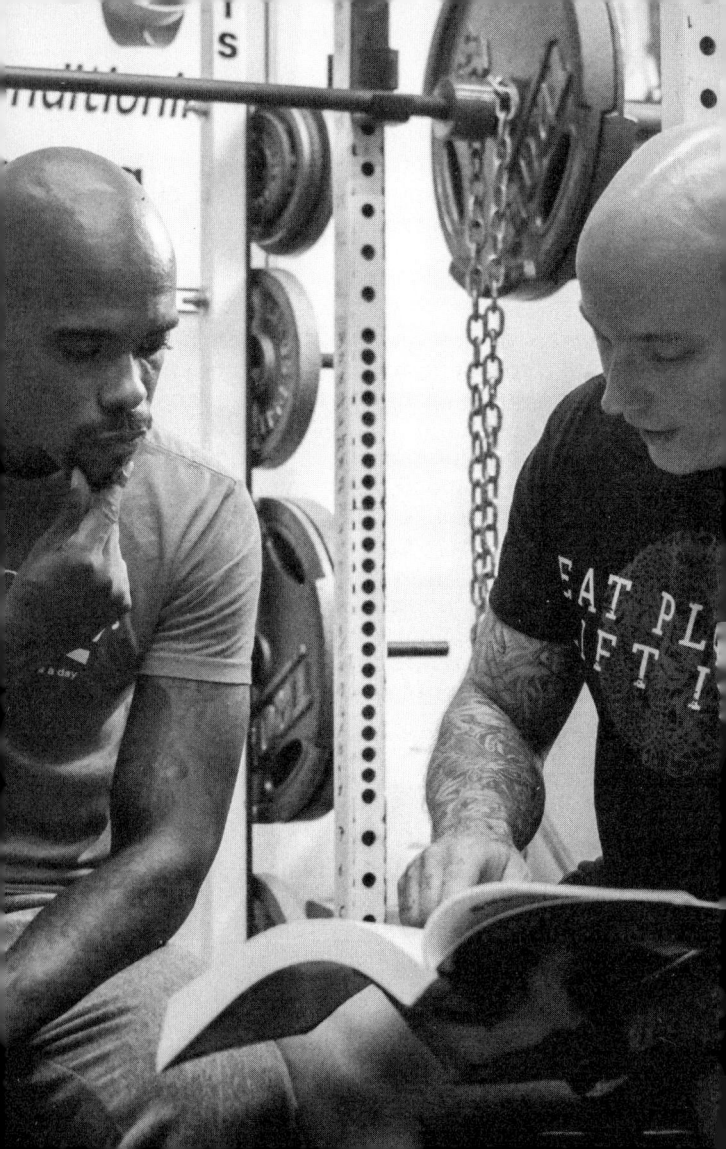

CHAPTER 3
BULKING: GERMAN VOLUME TRAINING

"Pump up the volume!"
- RAKIM

Once Scott had gotten enough preliminary data and calculated the numbers, he told me that we are going to move into the bulking phase of the program he had in mind for me and after that we would move into a cutting phase. So we would build up my weight and muscle first and then chisel and define it next. Scott said that for the bulk phase I would be lifting to make the biggest gains in our experiment. He said I would have to shovel down food like a forklift and lift a gang of weight. He introduced me to the concept of German Volume Training (GVT) that was made famous by Charles Poliquin. Scott breaks it down to the nuts and bolts later but it's pretty much where you do a shit load of reps and multiple sets like in the 100 reps range. It's a super intense approach. It felt like some kind of boot camp for weight lifting to me but I soldiered up.

WHOLE BODY STRENGTH

Scott set my training week up so I would be hitting ALL my major muscle groups consistently, so I could

THE STUDENT IS READY

gain all around strength and not just cosmetic "beach muscles". We weren't going to just be working out the upper body, biceps and chest on Scott's watch. Scott wanted me to have a solid foundation in real weight training and he insisted on a well-rounded approach to developing my size and strength.

TECHNIQUE

That German Volume Training was insane enough but on squat day, the shit was bonkers. On squat day it seemed like a huge mountain that I'd be coming in to climb. Scott taught me how to breathe through that intensity though. He taught me to suck in my air, take a full deep breathe and hold it and then set up evenly under the squat bar. Put the bar right on the top of my back and squeeze my shoulder blades together. Then while holding that air in like a tight compressor, I'd lift the bar out of the rack and squat down as parallel as I could and sit back into the bench, then breathe out as I push from my heels through to my hams and quads into my lower back and up for one rep and then repeat.

Scott would be yelling to encourage me "Stay tight!" And remind me to mind my form and it really helped me to focus into what I was doing. In between some of the maniac amounts of GVT reps Scott would also have me doing "super sets" of pull-ups for multiple sets, then after that I'd see how many pull-ups I could do until failure.

Call me crazy, but I was loving it! I loved that sore feeling the day after a hard session. I was starting to get positively addicted to the Iron.

> *"Some are body builders*
> *Some are power lifters*
> *I'm just becoming an iron man*
> *Bar-mitzvah*
> *Sweat pouring libation like a bartender*
> *But I'm thinking big like Giant from the Bartendaz*
> *Blame it on the comic book ads when we was shorties*
> *Beach girls like big dudes, but if you scrawny*
> *They kick beach sand in ya face Man it was lonely*
> *Looking at my ribs in the mirror it made me hungry*
> *Feed me iron, from a skinny cat into lion*
> *Strong and lean like the Mayans*
> *I rep the hard gainers and ectomorphs*
> *Don't feel right til my chest is sore this is what I live for...*
> *Building my power base with core strength*
> *No short cuts, Just More pounds and more reps..*
> *A lifters brain is abnormal*
> *If I ain't sore from training I'm going thru withdrawal"*
> *-Stic*

EXTREME TEAM

As my training progressed I had the pleasure to meet some of Scott's other clients. Karl is a 6 1/2 foot super fit world-class swimmer with curly blond hair, whose

THE STUDENT IS READY

early morning personal training session with Scott often overlapped with mine. Really humble; cool guy. I'd watch him go through his regimen like a beast pushing and sweating and his focus and dedication was inspiring. I got to see how an advanced level competitive swimmer utilizes iron to enhance his game. He'd be sweaty and breathing heavy and wrapping up when I'd be walking through the door just getting ready to get started. Scott would take the time to explain to me some of the strategy behind why he had Karl doing certain exercises. Scott used the weights and other calisthenic combinations to simulate what Karl experiences at his competitive meets and explained how Karl's competitive performance would benefit from the drills and exercises he prescribed. It was amazing to see the brilliant strategies executed by Karl's champion-level of focus.

QUANTUM LEAPS

Then another of Scott's clients that I had the pleasure of meeting and training beside was Howard "Cosmonaut" Palmer. Cos keeps an immaculate Isaac Hayes styled beard, has a Jamaican-British English accent and a really positive and energetic spirit. He is an expert Parkour artist and stuntman. Parkour is a running sport that includes jumping, climbing and flipping and is based on developing the abilities for clearing obstacles with speed, balance, efficiency and finesse. To me it looks like a combination of sprinting, with the danger of mountain climbing and the creativity of break dancing all in one! Cosmonaut happened to be a fan of my music, too. His regimen was different than Karl's and I saw how Scott was able to cater his expertise to Cosmonaut's needs for the sport of Parkour. I'd see Cos doing amazing feats like jumping vertically what seemed to be like 5 or more feet high or jumping across the room in all sorts of "Spider man" type of skilful displays. I started to call him the Black Spider man. I got to watch many more of his amazing stunts, flips and jumps in videos online.

He had a serious injury to one of his arms and shoulder area that left it visibly weaker than the other and Scott helped him to train for re balancing his strength as well as improve his jumping and other areas. Cos is not only an incredibly inspiring Parkour artist, I was equally inspired by his philosophical approach to Parkour and his confidence and strength to rehabilitate his injury without letting it stop him. We have become buddies and we often go on group runs together.

Meeting these pros and some of Scott's other clients helped motivate me to want to maintain a high standard of dedication as well. I felt honored to be a part of the EXTREME Team and the spirit of dedicated training that Scott has established at Extreme Performance Training Systems.

THE STUDENT IS READY

IRON CULTURE INSPIRATION

We did weeks of GVT and it was super beast mode. I was loving it though! Scott was not only teaching me technique but also feeding me motivation by sharing knowledge on the Iron Culture.

LEGENDS OF THE IRON

Scott showed me some YouTube videos of this humongous tatted up, muscle bound Compton OG named CT Fletcher. This guy is an Iron Legend out of the world renowned Metroflex Gym in Long Beach California. He is hilarious and extremely motivating. Imagine the prolific profanity of Richard Pryor mixed with the personality of a gangsta-drill sergeant all blended up with a mean ass dad that you can still somehow sense the love within the tough tactics, and that's CT Fletcher. He is a sought after trainer and former world-class lifting competitor and also world push up champion too. His videos became part of my morning breakfast. There's no way you can be on your way to the gym and listen to CT and not feel ten times more amped to hit that iron with all you got! I found myself so inspired by his raw hard-core style and have been telling my comrades to follow him on social media for inspiration ever since.

Scott put me up on game about another legend in the world of physical culture named Steve Jeck. This guy is a giant in weight lifting, and stone lifting, literally, as well as a gifted writer and speaker. Scott told me one story about Jeck where Jeck is explaining his views on barbell training in a gym as compared to stone lifting in nature. Jeck says that a barbell is made to be lifted. It's balanced and has the nice little bar made to be gripped with the knurling grooves; essentially it has been crafted and designed to be lifted. He goes on to say but the stone doesn't help you lift it. It's unbalanced, hard to hold and resists being easily moved about. Lifting stones, Jeck proclaims builds a greater more natural and functional kind of strength. The distinction he makes is that barbells are heavy, while stones are defiant! He has a great audio CD called Classic Jeck with essays on strength development in mind and body that he wrote and reads aloud. His powerful baritone voice sounds like Zeus speaking and his ideas are heavily motivational.

Then there is Henry Rollins, a true Rock star and a true lifter. Scott is a huge fan of The Rollins Band as the posters around the training center attest to. Scott shared with me that Rollins was a man of the Iron as well and as a musician that is into fitness I found that doubly inspiring and relatable. He would have Rollins Band music cranking as we trained and I started getting into it too. The lyrics are strong and clever and the music is energetic and edgy like you'd expect from rock but the way Rollins sings is kind of like poetry or old school rap, too.

THE STUDENT IS READY

Scott shared with me their album Weight, which featured an iron plate on the cover and he quoted from some of Henry's verse lyrics that seem to reflect some of his weight training. One favorite song is "On my way to the Cage" from the album Come in and Burn. As a producer, I'm into all kinds of music and I really appreciated this new find. Come to find out the Rollins Band bass player Melvin Gibbs worked with my group dead prez in several sessions in NYC back in the day. Small world.

Scott also shared with me this incredibly inspiring article that Henry Rollins wrote called The Iron that really inspired me and captured what I was starting to appreciate about my experiment with weight training. You can find it in its entirety online but here is a snippet:

"The Iron is the best antidepressant I have ever found. There is no better way to fight weakness than with strength. Once the mind and body have been awakened to their true potential, it's impossible to turn back.

The Iron never lies to you. You can walk outside and listen to all kinds of talk, get told that you're a god or a total bastard. The Iron will always kick you the real deal. The Iron is the great reference point, the all-knowing perspective giver. Always there like a beacon in the pitch black. I have found the Iron to be my greatest friend. It never freaks out on me, never runs. Friends may come and go. But two hundred pounds is always two hundred pounds" - **Henry Rollins, The Iron**

TRAINING MUSIC

Music played a big part of our sessions. We played my album The Workout probably 10,000 times! We also listened to a gang of other stuff to keep the energy flowing and the motivation up. Linkin Park, Jay Z and loads of Tech N9ne. Until I started training with Scott, I hadn't ever really took the time to appreciate Tech N9ne's lyrical creativity and just the pure dopeness of his production but I found it to be a supersonic boost that helped get me through some intense sessions.

Not only was my strength increasing, so was my awareness and appreciation of the Iron culture as well as my musical exposure was expanding.

FORKLIFT – FUELLING THE MACHINE

When I'd leave the gym it would be time to refuel. Scott told me I needed to start eating within 30 minutes or less after I finish my work out to optimize my efforts for growth. Based on Scott's suggestion, my wife Afya put me on a six meal a day plan; three big meals and two to three smaller ones.

I had to really prioritize my eating to make new habits because I'd been used to eating sporadically. The foods I was eating were healthy, mostly organic of course but my frequency and consistency of eating was random and inconsistent. Afya had me approach my dietary shift methodically.

EAT BIG BUT DON'T OVER DO IT

First, Afya had me understand that I needed to add about 500 more calories a day. She said I would have to eat more than I'm used to eating but it was important that I still not OVER eat. She said a big tendency people who want to gain weight is to think they can just eat as much as they want, the more the better, but that wasn't healthy or effective. Afya explained to me that the body can only process so many calories a day and too many calories would only stress the body and create unhealthy and unsightly complications. She echoed what Scott had also said that the goal is to give the muscles enough extra calories to rebuild but if we over did it the excess beyond what was necessary would be stored as fat.

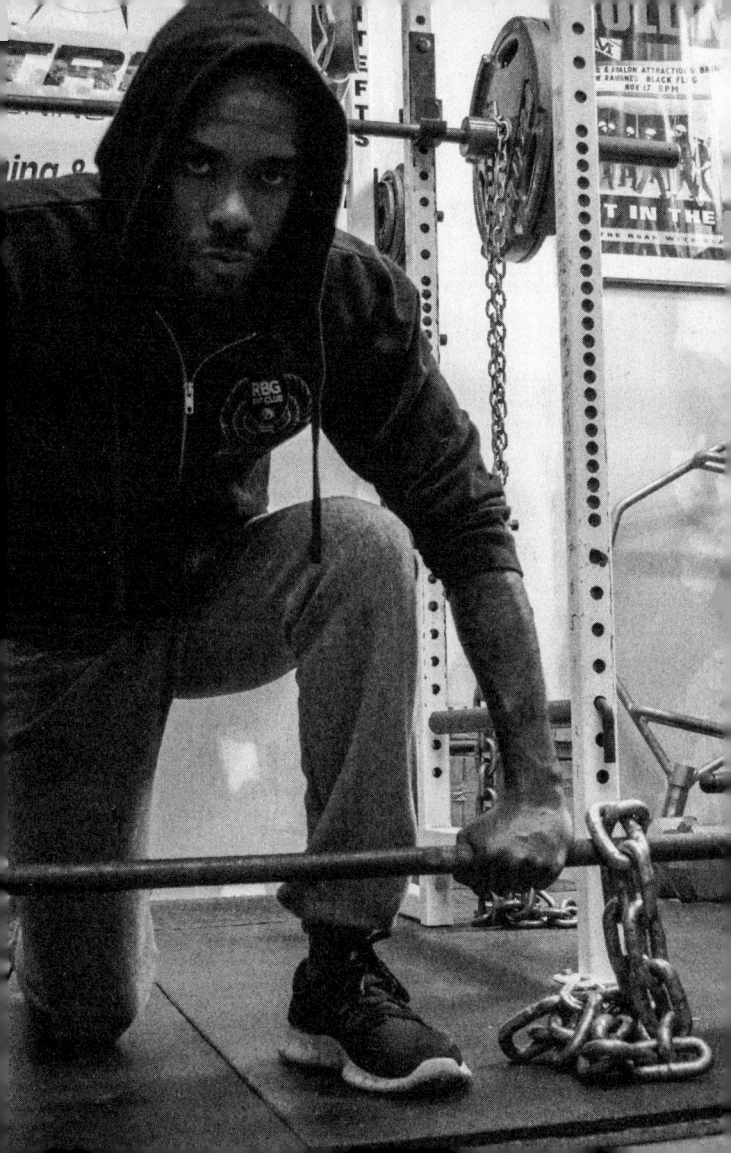

THE STUDENT IS READY

GUACAVELI
(Stic's Original Recipe)
Yield 2 Cups

Ingredients
2 Organic Hass Avocados
1 Small onion, finely chopped
1 Ripe tomato, chopped
1 Lime, juiced
1/4 Cup of fresh chopped cilantro
Sea salt and red pepper flakes to taste

Directions:
1. Peel avocados in a medium serving bowl. Add chopped onion, cilantro, tomato. Mash until creamy blend develops but still chunky. Squeeze in lime juice, and mix in sea salt and red pepper to taste. Chill for half an hour to blend flavors.

Nutrients per serving:
Calories 122
Fat 9g
Carbs 11g
Protein 3g

IRON VEGAN WEIGHT GAIN SHAKE 700+ CALORIES.

1 Banana
1 cup Hemp Milk
½ cup Raw Pumpkin Seeds
3 tbsp Flaked Coconut (Unsweetened)
1 Cup Blue Berries
1 tsp, Ginger root - Raw
1 cup Filtered Water
¼ cup Agave Nectar or maple syrup
2 tbsp Peanut Butter-no Salt, Unsweetened
2 tsp Wheat Grass Powder

Steps:
1. Fill powerful blender about half way with water
2. Drop in all ingredients and blend till smooth
3. Makes about 32oz
4. Lasts about 6 -8 hours refrigerated

Nutrients per serving
Calories 898
Fat 39g
Carbs 123g
Protein 26g

THE STUDENT IS READY

STIC'S 10 MINUTE STIR FRY

Ingredients:	Nutrients per serving
1 tbsp Sesame oil	Calories 201
1/2 cup Red bell pepper	Fat 10g
2 tsp Minced garlic	Carbs 19g
3 cups Spinach	Protein 9g
1 can Chickpeas	
1/2 tsp Sea salt	
1/2 tsp Smoked paprika	
1/4 tsp Onion powder	
Squeeze of lemon juice	

Directions:
1. Add enough Sesame oil to lightly cover large sauce pan
2. Turn on heat to medium
3. Wash and Slice organic red bell pepper and add to pan
4. Add a few Teaspoons of minced garlic (I like a lot)
5. Don't let it get dark brown before you add the spinach
6. Rinse 5 handfuls of baby
7. Spinach
8. Add to pan
9. Stir spinach around in oil garlic and red bell pepper for approx. 2min
10. Add a can or carton of organic chickpeas aka garbanzo beans
11. Season with roasted paprika
12. Sea salt onion powder and fresh lemon juice

STIC'S AR-15 APPLE RAISIN AND PEANUT BUTTER SNACK (MAKES 1 SERVING)

Two organic apples
1/8 cup organic raisins
3 tbsp Organic unsweetened peanut butter
Pinch of Cinnamon

Directions:
1. Slice the apples in approx. 1/8 inch thick chip like slices
2. Spread peanut butter on the apple slices
3. Sprinkle the raisins evenly on the peanut butter cover apple slices
4. Sprinkle on a Pinch of Cinnamon to taste

Calories 435
Fat 33g
Carbs 15g
Protein 16g

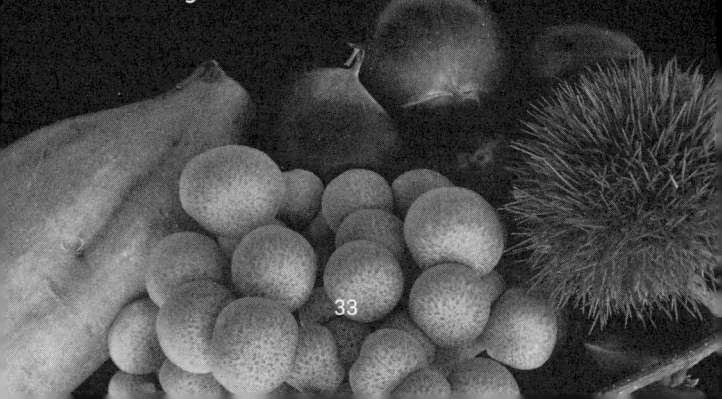

THE STUDENT IS READY

FOOD JOURNAL

Afya had me keep a daily food journal and I wrote down everything I ate and drank for weeks keeping a record so we could go back and look and see what was working or not and make adjustments accordingly. I became a human forklift, shovelling down the food but staying mindful of Afya's tips.

PROTEIN

I didn't have any trouble getting my protein in. Afya would often make dinners with quinoa, which is a complete source of plant-based protein that the ancient Andean and Incan cultures first cultivated thousands of years ago. I made chickpeas and spinach a lot for my smaller meals. I made a lot of salads with organic sprouted soy veggie burger and raw pumpkin seeds.

PUMPKIN SEEDS IS THE BUSINESS

Pumpkin seeds were in just about everything I ate. They are like one of the "secret weapons" of whole plant based protein sources. When it comes to protein they pack a punch. Just ¼ of a cup of raw pumpkin seeds has like 9.5 grams of protein! If you compare the protein content in them pound for pound not only do they match up to the leading supplement powders, without the added sugars and processing they are also a fraction of the cost!

*"I'm in the kitchen
Yams everywhere
Just left the gym
Feeling like a hungry bear
Garbanzo beans, Sautéed Kale
Getting my weight up heavyweight on the scale
Hell yeah I cook I'm not just a rapper
But my wife is Top Chef got me one like Padma
Pantry stockpiled like an army bunker
I'm trying to be on my Vin Diesel by the summer
I lift the weight
Then I lift the fork
Stacking plates
Drinking big smoothies by the quart
This how I build the fort
Rock solid foundation
Stay disciplined
Follow through with dedication"
-Stic*

LESS FARTING IS ALWAYS GOOD

Afya taught me that the protein in seeds is easily broken down and digested within the body and I noticed I didn't have that heavy "itis" feeling when I would finish a plant based meal even though I was getting in loads of protein. I also noticed I wasn't having all the farting that comes with shovelling down all those expensive protein powders. What a relief that was for the fam!

THE STUDENT IS READY

PORTION CONTROL REMINDERS

Afya constantly coached me on quality ingredients and taught me how to eyeball portion sizes so I would reach my daily calorie goals but not over do it. I'd be just piling up my plate cause' I'm "trying to get big" and Afya was on point and reminded me that men have a tendency to think the bigger the better but that it's discipline and control that are the more efficient and effective ways to accomplish goals.

TWEAKING THE PLAN TO SUSTAIN ENERGY

At the same time, since I was also running distances of 6-10 miles a few times a week, she calculated that extra energy expense and made sure my caloric needs were adjusted and met on those days too. She helped me to realize that if I ate consistently I'd have enough energy for the high-energy demands I was asking my body to sustain for this experiment. I also enjoyed drinking my home brewed 5 Elements Tea on my running days for an extra boost of natural energy.

> **STIC'S 5 ELEMENT ENERGY TEA**
>
> Organic Yerba Mate Tea bag (fire)
> Organic Peppermint Tea bag (air)
> 20oz hot Water (water)
> 1 Cup Hemp milk (earth)
> ¼ Tsp Raw Agave optional for taste (metal)

WATER LOG

A big challenge was getting in enough of the recommended amounts of water each day while having to consume all that food. She said that I would need to drink a minimum of half my body weight in ounces everyday. So starting at 167lbs meant I had to throw back at least around 85 ounces of H2O a day plus extra when I run. My stomach would be full as the evening tide but I spaced it out in between snacks and meals and made it happen as close as I could every day.

Afya "drink water" Ibomu is kind of like a hydro maniac promoter of hydration but I mean that in a good loving way.

Afya explained that drinking all that water was so important to my gains because it helped my body transport the protein to my muscles efficiently and it kept me flushed, hydrated and running smoothly. I split my daily water quota up using my trusty 26oz RBG FIT

THE STUDENT IS READY

CLUB stainless steel water bottle. I knew if I drink one when I wake up, one midday, one in the evening and one close to bed time, I'd have gotten in over 100 ounces for the day. Of course, the water goddess said the extra wouldn't hurt. Afya's great hydration habits have been a positive influence on mine. This woman literally sleeps with her water bottle! But her skin is flawless and she literally still looks like the same or even healthier 18 year old that I met over 20 years ago.

THE IRON STRENGTHENS BALANCE

I was getting into the rhythm of my regimen and it was feeling like a well-oiled machine that helped to structure my days with purpose. Prioritizing this intensive regimen of training with my other responsibilities as a husband, father, CEO, hip hop artist, producer, writer, son and social activist forced me to be more organized. I actually became more productive and started to get a lot more accomplished because of the heightened focus the lifestyle required.

LIFTER'S HIGH

I liked how the balance of my running days and my weight training days started to compliment each other. I noticed if I did a long run on a Tuesday and then went in with Scott and did a leg day with a gang of squats on Wednesday, the squats would actually seem easier than if I didn't run. I could also see that like the runner's high that I feel when I'm out there banging the miles out, I was starting to experience a kind of "lifter's" high when I get that pumped up feeling. I started to really crave that tight muscular soreness I'd feel after an intense iron workout.

I was really loving my experiment with the iron, but it ain't my day job. I'm a hip-hop artist and a main aspect of my livelihood is of course moving the crowd. I didn't want to lose my gains and slow my momentum but my regimen was interrupted several times by my touring obligations.

THE STUDENT IS READY

CHAPTER 4
MAINTAINING ON THE ROAD

"Ninety-nine percent of the failures come from people who have the habit of making excuses."
- GEORGE WASHINGTON CARVER

I had constant shows where I'd be in an out of town that could have thrown my regular training schedule off without proper planning and discipline.

DISCIPLINE IN DENMARK

I was invited to be an Ambassador for Sustania. org to speak and perform live at their annual awards conference in Copenhagen, Denmark. Sustania.org is the world's leading sustainable technology innovation platform where companies, foundations and thought leaders come together to support and work with a tangible approach to sustainability. With a focus on readily available solutions, Sustainia's mission is to mature markets and sectors for sustainable products and services. The work of Sustainia equips decision makers, CEOs and citizens with the solutions, arguments, visions, facts and network needed to accelerate sustainable transformation in sectors, industries and our everyday life. Scott gave me a regimen to do in the hotel via Google docs to sustain my training while I attended the Sustania conference.

THE STUDENT IS READY

Wifey and I had to pack a gang of food for the long flight in order to stay on my eating every two hours routine. My son came along as well. We had to travel to Paris overnight then arrive in Denmark the next day. I hit the hotel Gym the following morning and trained while listening to Brian Tracy's No Excuses: Power of Self Discipline audio book.

LOSING THE WORKOUT, GAINING AWARENESS

A crazy thing happened while I was in the hotel attempting to turn on my computer to rehearse for the Sustania show; my computer crashed! I lost all the music I had been working on for the Workout 2! Gone. Ethered. That crash set me back on completing the album by a long shot. I took it on the chin and accepted that the Universe knows best and it must be something even better that the way has been cleared for it to be created. Thankfully I had previously sent the Sustania coordinators the performance tracks and was still able to rock the show.

The presentations were all sorts of leaders in the fields of science, agriculture, technology, business and environmental activism and their insights were enlightening, engaging and compelling. I learned 30% of the species on the planet are endangered due to corporate pollution of the environment. One professor who is a leading researcher on climate change noted the startling fact that the Earth has lost over 70 of its rivers in just the past 100 years.

I made a lot of powerful connections that night with various eco industry bankers, investors and even chopped it up about gangsta rap with the former CEO of Proctor and Gamble!

I hit the steam room daily while in Denmark and banged my workouts in the hotel gym early before the day would get underway. The steam was a great treat. My body needed it and it was well appreciated.

HITTING THE IRON IN THE OUTBACK

Another challenge to my regular training schedule with Scott came when dead prez had an Australian tour scheduled for New Years and so I was going to be away on the road for the ten days. I didn't know if I would be able to stay consistent with my training because of travel and time constraints. I also brought my wife and son with me to have some hang out time together and so I had to make a game plan that included chill time with them but also as to not lose all my progress in my weight regimen. I Google'd ahead to find the gyms in or near my hotel and Afya got her Google on to find health food stores and vegan friendly restaurant options in surrounding areas. I was able to find quality gyms and get my sessions. I also got some time to do a few yoga classes and get a few runs in on the beach. It can be a lot of work at times being

THE STUDENT IS READY

a touring artist while maintaining a holistic health and fitness lifestyle but I'm blessed to be able to be living my dreams doing what I want to be doing and challenging my self to keep reaching new levels.

NUMBERS DON'T LIE CHECK THE SCOREBOARD

After weeks in, my experiment with Weight lifting became very fulfilling and something I really looked forward to on my training days. I was learning about a whole new world and I could feel myself getting stronger each week. Pounds were adding up consistently and in just less than two and a half months, I got on the scale and I had already gone from 167lbs to 187lbs!

In pictures it started to be obvious to me that I had actually gained twenty pounds. My pants and shirts were getting a bit young. I could definitely see that my thighs and arms and chest had expanded noticeably. As I looked at myself in the mirror I could even see a little more fullness developing in my face. I had reached my weight gain goal of adding on twenty pounds in less than half of the time that we had aimed for, on a plant based, gluten free supplement free diet while running long distances! I saw first hand how much discipline and consistency it took. But with that twenty pounds I noticed something extra that I hadn't anticipated. A gut.

F GYM   ORD D

132	148	165		242	27
COHN	ROHN	ALINDO	ZER	BALICKI	BAU
365	185	42	150	505	57
COHN	ACOUN		HETER	BALICKI	
31				365	4
				BAL	

CHAPTER 5
MAKING THE CUT (AND SHAKING THE GUT)

"If you can't handle me when I'm bulking, you don't deserve me when I'm cut."
- MARILYN MONROE

It's funny how when you get what you wish for it doesn't always turn out how you thought it would be. I was happy that the scale showed that I was 20lbs up, but I was uncomfortable with this new stomach I had developed. Scott told me not to worry about it. He said it was normal to add on some amount of fat during the bulking phase. He said that it was inevitable but that during the next phase of our program we'd cut it up in no time.

Afya also encouraged me and tried to help me realize that this was just a part of the process. She said as we shift into the cut phase, the dietary routine would also shift to assist the cutting process and help me lean up.

CUT BACK ON CALORIES

Afya cut back my calories by about 10 percent I think and that was tough for me. I had gotten used to eating mega amounts of food and it had become easy to do. Food is chemicals and those chemical proportions

THE STUDENT IS READY

and dosages become like "drugs" when we get used to certain amounts regularly. I noticed how having to be even more mindful of how much of something I was eating started to make me feel somewhat tense and uptight. I noticed how I would get irritated when Afya would remind me that I couldn't have a certain oil or vegan pastry dessert or as much rice or noodles as I wanted to eat because of how those fats and carbs would work against the goal of the cut phase.

ON THE ROAD AGAIN

Another UK tour came up for dead prez. For this tour there was hardly any gym access to be found. My comrade DivineRBG, who also hits the gym heavy, toured with us and helped out with the merchandising. He and I were on the constant hunt for gyms because the hotels we were staying in didn't have those accommodations.

MAKING IT DO WHAT IT DO

We also had a gruelling daily travelling schedule doing one show a day in a new city for 12 days straight, no days off. So D and I made due by using our luggage as barbells and doing body weight calisthenics in the hotel rooms. We ran our miles around the city to find vegan food options and we took care of business. I had to settle for less than organic on most occasions and I ate more than my share of fries and falafels but hey, shows got rocked, training got done and basic goals got met. It wasn't ideal but it was better than no training at all. By the time I got back I could tell my progress was affected.

FEELING OFF

I got off the road and got right back into the regular swing of things with Scott and doing my distance runs but I felt kind of "off". I was kind of feeling like I was behind. On the road I had lost some of the sense of dedication being that I had to adjust and make due with what was available training and diet wise.

I noticed I started to slack on my strict adherence to the game plan of the dietary restrictions. I kind of justified it by saying I'm going to eat a little more carbs cause I was on the road and I probably need to make sure I replenish those missed calories.

I had lost a few pounds and was kind of worried that I might have reversed a lot of my hard work while on tour. We were in like the 5th month or so of training and balancing of all my responsibilities personal and professional became more challenging. I saw my focus starting to weaken a bit as daily life's anxieties, sleep challenges, touring, and the extended duration of the experiment started taking its toll.

THE STUDENT IS READY

ELITE INSPIRATION

One of Afya's other clients at the time was a fitness competitor bikini model and Afya would tell me how meticulously disciplined those high-level competitors diets are. I learned how every gram of proteins, carbs, fats and even salt was measured out to a strict ratio and adhered to unfailingly. I was humbled in my realization that the competitive fitness lifestyle is an extremely disciplined path requiring tremendous dedication and self-control and I see why only the elite are able to maintain their champion levels of athleticism over the long haul.

A friend of ours happens to be one such elite competitor.

Torre "Tha Vegan Dread" Washington is the epitome of Vegan Bodybuilding. He has been a vegetarian since birth, vegan for the last 16 years, and is one of the top champion vegan bodybuilders in the entire sport. Dude is ridiculously diesel and defined and is a really focused and inspiring human being.

Afya and I met Dread at the Atlanta Veg Fest one year and have been friends for a while now. He and Afya tag team counselling fitness competitor clients where he provides the training and she provides the nutritional guidance. Afya showed me her client's super strict food regimen for motivation. Afya helped her to transition to a plant based lifestyle and her client went on to win first place in her pro bikini competition! I was humbled and needed to put my little experiment in perspective. I realized if I was going to honor the process, I needed to hang in there and get my focus back. But it was hard to ignore the extra roundness poking out under my T-shirt.

THE STUDENT IS READY

CHAPTER 6
GO HARDER

"No citizen has the right to be an amateur in the matter of physical training... What a disgrace it is for a man to grow old without ever seeing the beauty and strength of which his body is capable"
- SOCRATES

The aim of the cut phase was to keep as much of the weight and muscular gains as possible while lowering my body fat percentage by as much as possible. Scott shifted my strength training focus from heavy weight centered strength gains to a higher rep, cardio type of focus. Kettle bell swings, loads of abs work and this heavy sled that football players use called The Prowler. He also suggested that I maintain my distance runs and add some sprint days as well.

TURN UP

As my training intensified with more reps, more ab work and more cardio, still my gut was stubborn, so we turned the intensity of my training up a few more notches. After my regular weight training work for the day Scott started to have me use the Prowler.

THE STUDENT IS READY

ON THE PROWL

We'd go out back in the parking lot. I would do 5 set rounds. In a descending pyramid pattern I would start with 25 kettle bell swings then push the Prowler 50 yards out and 50 yards back across the surface of the concrete, then rest for a minute or so. Then repeat the whole circuit with 20 swings and repeat the prowler push. Then 15. Then 10, then 5.

I'd also do this ab circuit where I do 25 kettle bell swings then three types of weighted abs exercises like crunches, twisting sit ups and leg lifts on the floor for 25 reps each. I'd do that in the same descending pattern from 25 to 20 to 15 to 10 to 5 with the 3-part abs circuit as super sets in between the kettle bell sets.

STEP UP THE RUNNING

If it happened to be my distance run day or sprints day I'd leave Extreme Performance Training Systems and then go bang out some miles as well. My buddy Sheik and I often do regular runs together and so I started inviting him on my sprint days too. Sometimes we would sneak in and run the steps of this outdoor stadium downtown. Other times we'd do 100 yard x 10 sprints in parking lots. Burning fat was the mission and I was training my ass off to cut the gut.

MEASURE OF A MAN

Scott took my body mass index measurements to see what progress we were making and my fat ratio was still more than I desired. I was becoming more frustrated because by this time it had been about 6 months of intense training day in and day out, super strict dietary regimen, super early bed times and I was getting to the point where I wanted to just be done with the whole experiment. I was losing faith in the process and I knew I was at the edge.

The cut phase of my experiment was definitely the toughest phase physically but more so mentally. It forced me to face the fragility of my patience, the shakiness of my faith and to question the integrity of my determination.

NOT MYSELF

The restrictiveness of the "cut" phase diet seemed like it had been dragging on too long and frankly I was tired of it. When I was just stuffing food down in the bulk phase I got used to that quickly and liked it and it became routine but the cut phase diet seemed like a nagging force of can'ts and don'ts. I don't know if it was some kind of withdrawal symptoms from the chemical in all the carb heavy foods I had gotten used to eating but my optimist attitude was turning sourpuss.

THE STUDENT IS READY

Sometimes I ate some carbs even when I knew I wasn't supposed to. Then I'd feel like such a slacker. Them carbs is the devil, I thought. My wife jokingly started calling me Aretha Franklin, because like in the Snicker's commercial when they say "you are not yourself when you are hungry" and the hungry cranky guy in the back seat turns to Aretha Franklin, well that was me.

MOMENT OF TRUTH

One day my wife and I were parked in front of Whole foods about to grab some groceries and I expressed my frustrations to her. Thankfully, she is skilled as a holistic health counsellor at helping clients work through their challenges. She listened and encouraged me not to give up and to give it a bit more time while she formulated the missing piece of the puzzle.

"If you always put limits on everything you do, physical or anything else, it will spread into your work and into your life. There are no limits. There are only plateaus, and you must not stay there, you must go beyond them." - BRUCE LEE

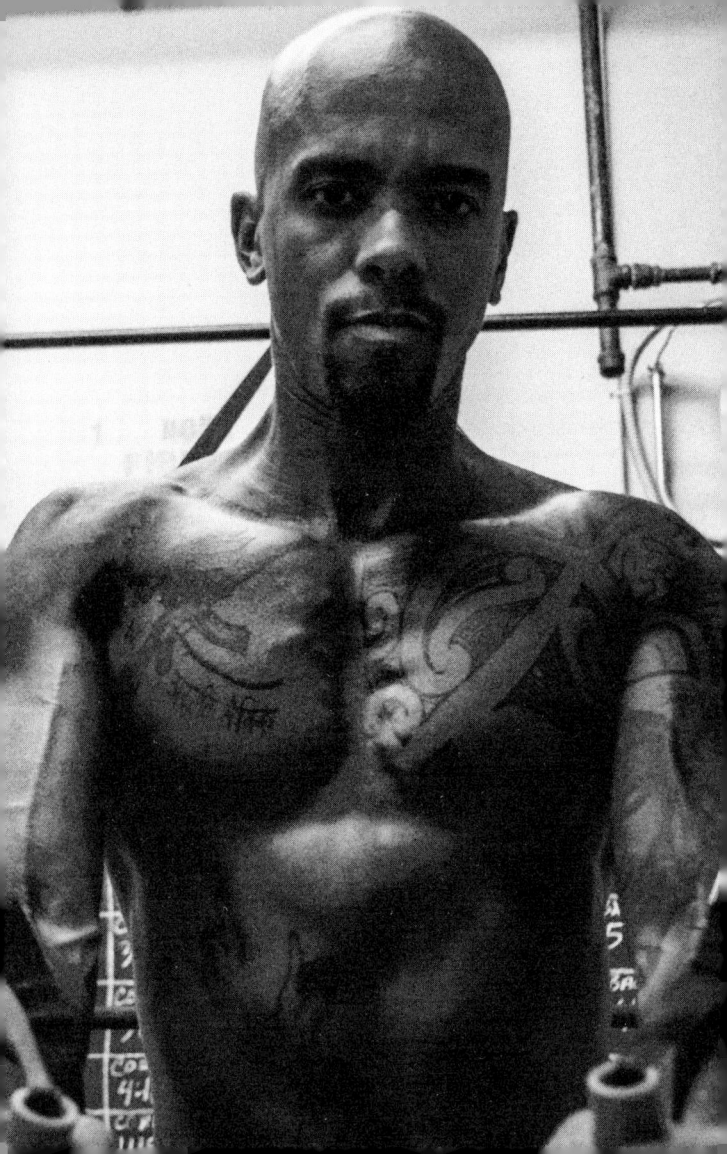

CHAPTER 7
LEAN BULK

"I saw the Angel in the marble and carved it until
I set him free"
- MICHELANGELO

Afya did her research and came up with a strategy to adjust my "cutting" diet to a more lean bulking approach. Lean bulking is where you still get in your big calories but what you eat is "clean", essentially minimizing processed foods and fat consumption. With the lean bulking approach I would be able to maintain my gains and eat more options of foods that I enjoyed. I increased my water intake and my cardio and I could have some oil in my meals, some carbs but within a ratio that Afya figured out that would minimize the retention of the fat.

WINNER MENTALITY

The lean bulking shift came right on time. I felt like I had more options and I felt more positive about finishing my training experiment and giving it all I got the last couple of weeks. I ran consistently, stuck to Afya's dietary guidelines and I hit a dead lift PR of 305lbs shortly after!

THE STUDENT IS READY

TEAM PLANT BUILT

Scott and I had agreed to wrap up the experiment right around the time we were all going to Austin, Texas for the 2014 Naturally Fit Games. Scott was competing as a member Team Plant built's power lifting squad. Plant Built is a vegan muscle team of 31 professional and amateur strength and fitness competitors, including Robert Cheeke one of the modern day founders of the Vegan Bodybuilding movement. Giacomo Marchese, founder of Plant built asked me to attend the games as a guest and to perform at the Plant built team's after party. Scott and I decided that would be a great time to bring our experiment to a close, tally our findings and celebrate what we accomplished.

CHAPTER 8
REACHING BIGGER GOALS

"Slowly getting bigger, I'm seeing definition
Flexing in the mirror my pecs getting thicker
Squats got my calves and my quads on sizzle
My abs getting chiselled, I've been on my grizzle
I'm loving my training; I'm always on it
Cause I'm building up the body that I always wanted"
-Stic

I pushed through the last weeks of training with all I had. When we did our final measurements and calculations I felt stronger than ever. I weighed 180lbs and my body fat percentage had dropped lower than it was at the start of the experiment. I could see my abs had made their comeback and I felt empowered and grateful.

I thoroughly enjoyed the Eat Plants, Lift Iron experiment. I proved to myself I could do it even though at times I wanted to quit. With skinny genetics, a super high metabolism, tall, long narrow thin limbs and frame, on a plant based diet, while long distance running and travelling, using no protein powders, gluten or tree nuts, I was able to gain 20lbs of weight and significant amount of muscle and end off with a low body fat percentage.

THE STUDENT IS READY

I had come through months of intense training that pushed me to my edge physically and mentally. I had tested my focus and determination with the help of two great experts guiding me and helping me forward. I learned many lessons about strength and discipline and hard work and consistency. I experienced the power of mind over matter.

TAKE AWAYS

I saw that with teamwork and the power of the willing mind and a determined spirit; the body can be shaped into the vision that you imagine. It inspired me not only that I can accomplish my goals in the gym but in life with that same focus and discipline. I think the biggest "gain" is beyond the great benefits of health and stamina, or the twenty pounds or even any of the PR's in strength that I hit. The big takeaway for me was a timeless jewel that I think anyone who has ever committed themselves to going to war on the battlefield of the Iron, can attest to:

The Iron teaches us how to overcome resistance.

TEN TAKEAWAYS

1. Accept yourself as is, always.
2. Vision: Be Specific when Goal Setting. You hit what you aim at.
3. Teamwork makes the dream work. Conspire with the right team to help reach your goal.
4. Focus: stay inspired and fuelled by an enthusiastic commitment to purpose. Use books, motivational speakers, vision boards etc. to help your inspiration stay potent.
5. Commitment gets you through the Crunch. Quitters never win, winners never quit. Stay reminded why you have your goal.
6. Humility allows growth. Expect to be humbled in order to change.
7. Measurements help show progress and where to adjust for victory. Be scientific, keep journals and records of your progress.
8. Adapt and Conquer. Whatever is blocking your progress accept it and rise to the occasion to overcome it.
9. Do the Work. If you cheat on the work you cheat yourself out of results.
10. Perseverance Pays with interest. Appreciate and Stay on the path, there's more to the journey than the destination.

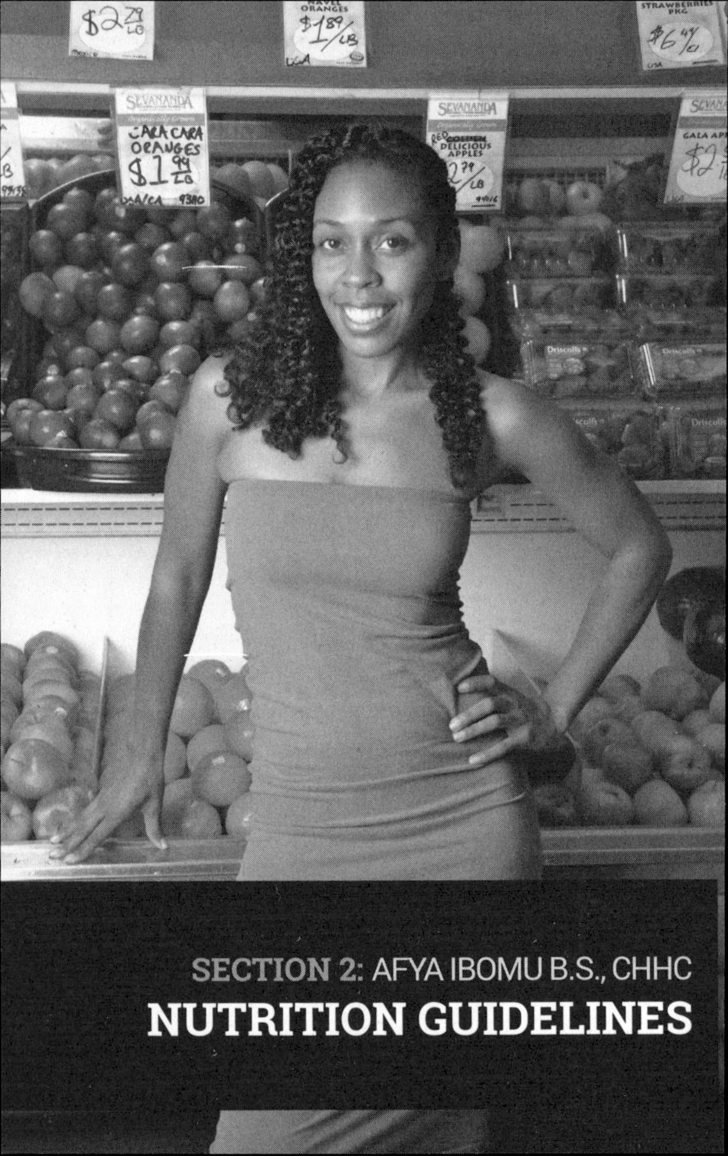

SECTION 2: AFYA IBOMU B.S., CHHC
NUTRITION GUIDELINES

CHAPTER 9
FEED THE FOCUS

"Just like keeping a healthy diet is important to maintaining a healthy lifestyle, eating the right foods is just as important for getting the most out of your workout."
- MARCUS SAMUELSSON,
MASTER CHEF

Being in a relationship with Khnum (Stic) for over 21 years I've seen his determination with working out and with different fitness challenges. Over the years, he has attempted a few times here and there to put on a bit more weight. He's tried using protein powders and performance enhancing natural supplements and even fish, to no avail. Each time he would gain a few pounds but then get symptoms of either over training or exhaustion or allergies and he would discontinue the program. Whatever small gains he had gotten would quickly fade and he would be back at his normal weight of about 165 pounds.

IRON CHEF

When Khnum told me that he wanted to try and gain weight and muscle with a plant based diet and not use any powders or performance supplements or fish, I was happy to help him make it happen. I'm not only

NUTRITION GUIDELINES

a nutritionist, I'm a chef and a hard-core foodie that's been plant based for 25 years so by default I'm sort of a hobby scientist and there is a part of me that loves to experiment, especially with food. Being plant based for so long I've heard all the questions and statements such as "where do you get your protein" or "you can't gain weight as a vegan" and the like. Questions like these are what motivated me to write my book The Vegan Soul food Guide to the Galaxy. So I was super hyped to be a part of this mission to document this process.

Khnum said he wanted the program to be more of a lifestyle than a diet and he wanted to be able to also continue running long distances, which is one of his passions. I knew he also has a sensitivity to gluten and tree nuts so we'd have to come up with all the nutrients he needed within those parameters as well. I began getting the strategy together with his trainer Scott.

BULKING & CUTTING: OUR NUTRITIONAL GAME PLAN

I like to work with trainers to get the maximum results. The trainers know what is generally needed to reach their clients goals, so I respect their input. Scott suggested that we use the approach of bulking and then cutting. This means gaining weight by first putting on the desired amount of pounds in both muscle and fat and then cutting the fat and sculpting the muscle.

HOLISTIC

As a holistic Nutritionist my role in this experiment was not only to create a balanced food plan that makes sure Khnum gets all the nutrients he needs and his daily quota of calories but also to make sure he is adequately hydrated and rested as well.

So now, let me explain how we approached Khnum's Bulk phase nutritionally in a bit more detail.

NUTRITION GUIDELINES

CHAPTER 10
THE INCREDIBLE BULK PHASE

> "I believe in fitness in it's entirety. The body is not the only thing important to great health, the individual has to be mentally prepared to maintain a healthy lifestyle."
> - JOHN 'BADASSVEGAN' LEWIS

During the bulk phase an increase in the amount of calories consumed each day is the primary goal to help build muscle and gain weight. We decided that Khnum's food intake should be to eat around six times daily. That would be three to four main meals a day plus 2-3 snacks. I was also working on a new cookbook at this time so he had full access to all of the desserts that I was making as well.

STIC'S BULKING MEAL PLAN

The following is a three day example of what Stic was eating and a breakdown of the nutrient intake during the Bulk phase.

NUTRITION GUIDELINES

DAY 1

BREAKFAST
1 Cup Gluten Free Quick Cooking Oats
1 Tblsp Raw Agave Nectar
4 Tblsp Hemp Seeds
2 Bananas
After workout Smoothie (Snack 1)
¼ Cup Raw Pumpkin Seeds
1 Cup Hemp Milk
2 Tblsp Peanut Butter, Unsweetened
1 Cup Blueberries
3oz Soy Yogurt
3 Tblsp raw agave nectar

LUNCH
1 Cup Rice noodles
4 Cups Tom Yum Vegetable Soup
Snack 2
20 Chips Blue Corn Chips
4 Tblsp Olive Hummus
1 Pear

DINNER
1 Large Baked Yam
2 Cups Bbq Tofu
¼ Cup Raw Pumpkin Seeds
1 Cup Kale cooked in Unsweetened Coconut Milk

SNACK 3 (Green Smoothie)
1 Cup Raw Kale
½ Cup raw Spinach
1 Apple
1 Pear

DAY 2

BREAKFAST
(Smoothie)
¼ Cup Blueberries
2 Tblsp Peanut Butter
1 Cup Hemp Milk
¼ Cup Pumpkin Seeds
2 Bananas
¼ Cup Boiled Sea moss
3 Tblsp raw agave

LUNCH (2 helpings)
1 Cup Organic Yellow Corn cheese Grits w/ Daiya Non dairy cheese
2 Gluten-Free Pancakes
1 Cup kale salad
6 Slices Coconut Curry Tempeh

SNACK 1
Avocado Cucumber Sushi Roll, 6pcs

DINNER
3 Cups Garden Vegetable Soup
2 Cups Quinoa

SNACK 2
2 Apples
4 Tblsp Peanut Butter, Unsweetened
¼ Cup Raisins

NUTRITION GUIDELINES

DAY 3

BREAKFAST
2 Tblsp Hemp Seeds
1 Large Baked Sweet Potato with skin
2 Cups scrambled tofu

SNACK 1 (Smoothie)
1 Banana
1 Pear
1 Cup Raw Spinach
1 Cucumber, with peel
2 Tblsp Hemp Seeds

LUNCH
1 Organic Sunshine Burger
1 Cup Black Beans
2 Tblsp Salsa
1 Cup shredded Lettuce
1/4 Cup Black Rice
4 Blue Corn Taco Shells

SNACK 2
4 Tblsp Olive Hummus
20 Blue Corn chips

DINNER
2 Gluten Free Sandwich Rounds
1 Qrunch Quinoa Burgers
2 Cups White Bean and Kale Soup

SNACK 3
1/3 Cup Dry Roasted Peanuts
¼ Raisins
4 Gluten free peanut butter cookies

The following displays the range of Stic's nutrients during the bulk phase. This was important for us to keep a track of so that we would know how to change his nutrients for the cut phase. As you can see all of his nutrients had a large range.

Calories: 2,890-3,666
Fat: 93-136g
Carb: 383-531g
Protein: 100-151g

TEMPEH VS TOFU

Tempeh is made from fermented whole soybeans. Due to the fermentation process, tempeh has more protein, calories, and is more digestible and overall is a more nutri¬tious alternative to tofu. Tofu is also made from soybeans. The soybeans are boiled, ground up and a calcium salt is added to keep it together and then it's formed into tofu cakes or blocks. Studies have shown that soy can mimic natural human estrogen which could have harmful effects when eaten in large quantities or more than 25g a day.

RESULTS OF THE BULKING PHASE

After about 2 ½ months Khnum had already reached his goal of gaining twenty pounds! We saw that with this eating plan and training regimen it was very easy for him to gain weight. Right away we dispelled the

NUTRITION GUIDELINES

myth that it's impossible to gain weight as a vegan, and without supplements because our results showed that it is possible and very easy!

However, with that added weight and muscle that he gained came a significant amount of belly fat that he was not happy with. Stic had a difficult time accepting the weight that he gained because a lot of it was in his gut! Scott said this is a normal part of the process, so we started the Cut phase.

CHAPTER 11
NO SHORT CUTS: THE CUT PHASE MEAL PLAN

"If you really want to do something,
you'll find a way; if you don't, you'll find an excuse."
- JIM ROHN

During the cut phase, a decrease in the amount of calories (food consumed) is the primary goal to lose fat, and get leaner. During this phase we made drastic shifts in what Khnum had being eating during the Bulk phase. We cut out all added oils and processed foods such as pasta, flour, etc...

As you can see in the following three day sample meal plan below, Stic's nutrients were dramatically cut.

NUTRITION GUIDELINES

DAY 1

BREAKFAST
¼ Cup Raw Pumpkin Seeds
1 Cup Gluten Free Quick Cooking Oats
1 Small Gala Apple
1 Tblsp Peanut Butter, Unsweetened

LUNCH
2 Veggie Hot Dogs
2 Cups Cauliflower & Peas
1 Cup Brown Rice
16oz Fresh Vegetable Juice: Apple, Spinach, Beet, and Kale

DINNER
2 Cups Indian-Style Curry With Potatoes, Cauliflower, Peas, and Chickpeas
1 Cup pan fried tofu
1 Cup Indian lentil soup
Snacks
1 ½ Cup Hemp Milk
1 Cup Raw Carrots
4 Tblsp Olive Hummus
2 sheets Roasted Laver Seaweed

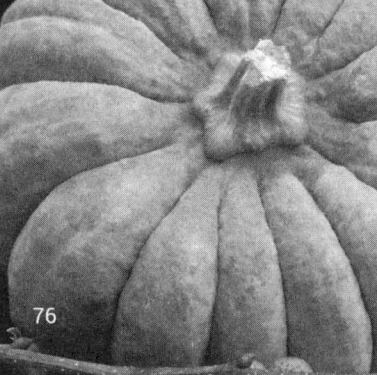

DAY 2

BREAKFAST
¼ Raw Pumpkin Seeds
1 Large Baked Large Sweet Potato
(Smoothie)
1 Banana
1 Cup Hemp Milk
2 Tblsp Peanut Butter Unsweetened
¼ Cup Blueberries
2 Tblsp Hemp Seeds

LUNCH
1 Cup Sprouted Tofu
2 Cups Kale sautéed
1 Cup Quinoa
16 oz Fresh Vegetable Juice: Apple, Spinach, Beet, and Kale

DINNER
8 oz Hemp Tofu
2 Cups Kale sautéed

SNACKS
¼ Cup Raisins
½ Cup Dry Roasted Peanuts
1 ½ Cup Hemp Milk
1 Apple

NUTRITION GUIDELINES

DAY 3

BREAKFAST
1 Tblsp Hemp Seeds
1 Small Gala Apple
1 Cup Gluten Free Quick Cooking Oats

LUNCH
1 Cup Brown rice
1 Cup Black beans
1 Cup shredded Lettuce
¼ Cup Tomato Pico De Gallo
3 Tblsp Guacamole
1 Cup Baked Tofu

DINNER
4 Veggie Hot Dogs
2 Cups garlicky green beans
2 Cups toss salad
16oz Fresh Vegetable Juice- Kale, Apple, Cucumber, Beet and Parsley

SNACKS
1 Apple
1 ½ Cup Hemp Milk
2 Tblsp Peanut Butter Unsweetened
4 Tblsp Olive Hummus
½ Cup Raw Celery
½ Cup Raw Carrots
2 Sheets Roasted Laver Seaweed

We cut Stic's nutrients about 15-20% to try and help cut his fat. During the Cut phase his daily nutrient intake ranged from:

Calories: 2270-2500
Fat: 60- 91g
Carb: 300-325g
Protein: 95-111g

CUT PHASE RESULTS:

After 5 months of this nutrition approach we cut his body fat by about 2% but it he was not happy with this process at all! He said the cut phase meal plan was too big on restrictions for such minimal results. He also went on a three-week tour as soon as we began the cut phase, which affected his ability to adhere to the cut meal regimen as precise as we would have liked. The limited amounts of carbs and fat were the most difficult for Stic, especially after he gotten used to being able to eat pretty much anything he wanted during the bulk phase. He was less enthused and becoming a bit frustrated with the process at this point, which I understood. We had to find a way for him to stay motivated and consistent on his regimen that would get the results we were after. I did more research and decided it might be our best bet to introduce the concept of lean bulking to our experiment.

NUTRITIONAL GUIDELINES

CHAPTER 12
GANGSTA LEAN

"Obstacles don't have to stop you. If you run into a wall, don't turn around and give up. Figure out how to climb it, go through it, or work around it."
- MICHAEL JORDAN

Meal planning for Lean bulking requires a much more precise approach than the bulking and cutting methods we were using. During the lean bulk phase the primary goal is to gain muscle while at the same time gaining the least amount of fat as possible. In lean bulking we are meticulously calculating and balancing several aspects of diet and training. We have to consider body fat percentage, ratios of macro nutrient amounts (calories, fat, protein, and carbs), the amount and type of exercise you do weekly and then we use a formula that guides the lean bulking strategy.

Lean bulking is one of the best ways to gain muscle with the least amount of fat and maintain the weight gain over time because when you're lean, you've got a revved-up metabolism and a body that wants to build muscle, not store fat. Keep in mind that everybody's needs are different and it takes experimenting with the calculations to figure out your exact macro nutrient needs for desired results.

NUTRITION GUIDELINES

CALCULATING MACRO NUTRIENTS

What are Macro nutrients: Macro nutrients are categories of foods that we need daily in large or "Macro" amounts. Protein, Carbohydrates and Fat are the macro nutrients we focus on in lean bulking and each contains a specific amount of calories that our bodies use for energy.

As stated earlier calculating the amount of macro nutrients you need is the basis to lean bulking. Each of us has an ideal mass/muscle building macronutrient profile. So it's not possible to make a blanket recommendation for the amounts of carbs, fats, and protein each person needs. But equations and calculations are a good place to start. Calculating macros may not be the most enjoyable thing to do but the extra effort will pay off big time, especially when you need to make adjustments in your nutrients down the road. When you know how much you eat each day, gaining or losing weight becomes a simple matter of math. There are many sites with calculators for you to input all of the info you need to figure out the amounts of macros you need based off your exercise routine. To make it easy I Google'd Lean Bulk Calculator and just entered the numbers they asked for (height, weight etc..) Keep in mind some calculators may ask you for body fat calculation but that number is not always necessary to get your macronutrient profile. Once I had his macronutrient profile I was able to use those numbers to come up with a meal plan.

I noticed that many calculators gave me a very high protein amount. Don't feel like you must reach that number daily! Please see the protein side note about the amount of protein needed daily. If you are using these calculators, keep in mind that they are just a guide. No one equation is 100% accurate but they allow you to have somewhere to start. Every 3-4 weeks you should track your weight and fat gain to see how the numbers are working for you then add or subtract from there.

Once I had Khnum's macronutrient profile, I organized his food plan using the website/app My Fitness Pal. I input his foods to correspond with his macro nutrients calculations and so that he would be eating every two hours. Due to his food allergies it was challenging to get all of his numbers exact while getting his food plan together. So I made considerations such as if his fat was a little high, his calories could be a little lower to balance out his intake amounts. As I said, these numbers are just estimates and they can be tweaked as you begin to see how your body responds.

NUTRITION GUIDELINES

LEAN BULK TIP*
Adjust your intake based on how your body is responding. If you are gaining too much body fat, drop your daily caloric intake by 250-500 calories. Likewise, if you find that you are not gaining weight after two weeks, increase your calories by 250-500.

TERMS TO KNOW

Here are a few terms that you will probably see when getting your macronutrient calculations:

Basal metabolic rate (BMR) is the minimum amount of energy the body needs to work or to sustain the body's essential metabolic processes. It is the number that represents the chemical interactions taking place in our bodies that provide the energy and nutrients needed to keep us alive. The BMR represents the energy the body uses while at rest and when a person just woke after an overnight fast.

THE THERMIC EFFECT OF FEEDING (TEF).
The TEF is the amount of energy used by the body after eating, in digesting and absorbing the nutrients from food and converting them for use or storage. TEF is usually assumed to be about 10-15% of the BMR, but is affected by a wide range of factors, such as

> the subject's nutritional status and the composition of the diet.
>
> **TEE THE TOTAL ENERGY EXPENDITURE**
> (Or TDEE) is the total of basal energy expenditure (BMR), the TEF and the amount of physical activity done daily/weekly. Increased activity raises the total, as does increased food intake (by increasing TEF).

STIC'S MACRONUTRIENT NEEDS

Here are stic's macro nutrient needs based off his unique calculations. As you can see his protein amounts vary greatly. There are many different thoughts about how much protein is really needed.

Calories = 2950
Protein = 90g - 130g
Carbohydrates = 385g
Fats = 73g
Water = 100+oz

Stic's daily nutrients from his lean bulk food plan ranged from:

Calories: 2736-2827
Fat: 87-97g
Carb: 382- 439g
Protein: 102-128g

NUTRITION GUIDELINES

7 DAY EXAMPLE OF STIC'S LEAN BULKING MEAL PLAN

DAY 1

BREAKFAST
24oz Water ½ before breakfast other half before lunch
Pre/post workout smoothie, 1 serving
1 Cup Yerba Mate tea with hemp milk and 1 Tblsp agave
1 Nectarine

LUNCH
2 Cups sautéed kale and tofu
2 Cups tossed salad with Papaya Poppy Seed Dressing
1 ½ Cup Quinoa
12oz Water
12oz coconut water

DINNER
3 Veggie Hot Dogs sautéed in veggie broth and garlic
1 Cup Quinoa
3 Cups Raw Spinach
24oz Water

SNACKS
1 Green smoothie
1 Cup Chamomile Tea with hemp milk and agave
3 Cups Watermelon
2 Tblsp Peanut Butter, unsweetened
1 Apple
24oz Water
2 Veggie Hot Dogs sautéed in veggie broth and garlic
3 Cups Raw Spinach

DAY 2

BREAKFAST
1/8 Cup Raw Pumpkin Seeds
1 Baked Sweet Potatoes including skin with 1 Tblsp maple syrup
1 Cup Yerba Mate Tea with agave and hemp milk
24oz water ½ before breakfast ½ before lunch

LUNCH
1 Cup Brown Rice
2 Cups kale and chickpeas
2 Sprouted Tofu Burgers
24oz Water

DINNER
1 Cup Brown Rice
6 Slices Coconut Curry Tempeh
2 Tblsp Hemp Seeds
2 Cups sautéed broccoli

SNACKS
Good morning1 (1 serving)
1 Cup Brown Rice
3 Slices Coconut Curry Tempeh
1 Cup sautéed broccoli
2 Cups Watermelon
1 Cup Chamomile Tea with agave and hemp milk
Water - Water Filter, 24oz

NUTRITION GUIDELINES

DAY 3

BREAKFAST
1 Cup Gluten Free Quick Cooking Oats with
1 Tblsp maple syrup
3 Tblsp Sesame seeds
1 small Apples
1 Cup Yerba Mate with hemp milk and agave
Water 24oz

LUNCH
2 Cups sautéed broccoli
1 Cup Brown Rice Penne Pasta
½ Cup Marinara sauce
2 Sprouted Tofu-Veggie Burgers
24oz Water

DINNER
2 Cups sautéed broccoli
1 Cup Brown Rice Penne Pasta
½ Cup Marinara sauce
2 Sprouted Tofu-Veggie Burger
24oz Water

SNACKS
1 Apple
2 Tblsp Peanut Butter, unsweetened
2 Veggie Hot Dogs sautéed with veggie broth and garlic
3 Cups Spinach
1 Cup Chamomile Tea with agave and hemp milk
24oz water

DAY 4

BREAKFAST
Good morning1 (1 serving)
Yerba Mate Tea with agave and hemp milk
Water 24oz

LUNCH
Moes - Burrito Bowl (Tofu, Black Olives, Rice, Black Beans, Peppers and Onions, Lettuce), 1 bowl
2 Tblsp Medium Salsa,
1 Peach
24oz Water

DINNER
2 Cups pan fried tofu
2 Cups sautéed broccoli
1 Cup Brown Rice
24oz Water

SNACKS
1 Cup pan fried tofu
1 Cup sautéed broccoli
1 Cup Brown Rice
3 Cups Watermelon
1 Cup Corn Flakes, Fruit Juice Sweetened
1 Banana
1/8 Cup Organic Thompson Raisins
1/3 Cup Raw Pumpkin Seeds
24oz Water

NUTRITION GUIDELINES

DAY 5

BREAKFAST
1 Baked Sweet Potatoes with skin and 1 Tblsp maple syrup
1 Cup Yerba Mate Tea with agave and help milk
24oz water half before breakfast and half before lunch

LUNCH
1 ½ Cups sautéed kale2
1 Cup pan fried tofu
1 Cup Brown Rice
1 Cup black beans
1 Peach
24oz Water

DINNER
1 ½ Cups sautéed kale2
1 Cup pan fried tofu
1 Cup Brown Rice
24oz Water

SNACKS
Snack smoothie, 1 serving
½ Cup Gluten Free Quick Oats with maple syrup
3 Tblsp Raw Pumpkin Seeds
2 Slices Corn Thins with 2 Tblsp Peanut Butter
2 Veggie Hot Dogs
3 Cups Watermelon
1 Cup Chamomile Tea with agave and hemp milk
24oz Water

DAY 6

BREAKFAST
Pre/post workout smoothie
1 Cup Yerba Mate Tea with hemp milk
And agave
24oz Water

LUNCH
1 Baked Sweet Potato with skin
2 Sprouted Tofu-Veggie Burgers
1 Cup sautéed broccoli
24oz Water

DINNER
2 Cups kale and chickpeas
1 Cup Brown Rice
1 Sprouted Tofu-Veggie Burger
1 Peach
24oz Water

SNACKS
3 Cup air-popped Popcorn with soy free margarine
1Cup Fruit Juice Sweetened - Corn Flakes in hemp milk
1/8 Cup Raisins,
1 Banana
1 Cup Chamomile Tea with agave and hemp milk
24oz Water

NUTRITION GUIDELINES

DAY 7

BREAKFAST
1 Cup Gluten Free Quick Cooking Oats with maple syrup and 1 Tblsp Sesame seeds
1 Apple
1 Cup Yerba Mate Tea with hemp milk and agave
24oz Water

LUNCH
1 Cup garlicky green beans
1 Cup Chickpeas
1 Cup Brown Rice
1/8 Cup Raw Sunflower Seeds
1 Peach
24oz water

DINNER
2 Cups tossed salad with 2 Tblsp Papaya and Poppy seed Dressing
½ Cup chickpeas
3 Veggie Hot Dogs
1/8 Cup Raw Pumpkin Seeds
24oz Water

SNACKS
Good morning1, (1 serving)
Green smoothie 2, (1 serving)
3 Cups air-popped Popcorn with soy free margarine
3 Cups Watermelon
1 Cup Chamomile Tea with agave and hemp milk

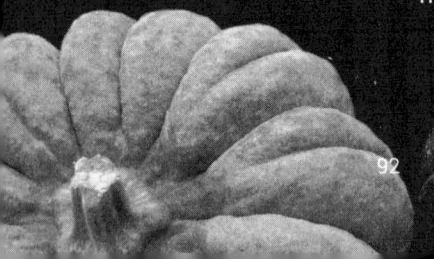

GANGSTA LEAN GROCERY LIST

PROTEIN
Organic Sprouted Tofu
Tempeh
Beans
Veggie hot dogs/burgers

CARBS
Quinoa
Wild Rice
Brown rice
Gluten Free Oats
Corn
Brown rice tortillas
Corn tortillas
Vegetables
Fruits
Brown rice noodles
Sweet Potatoes

FATS
Avocado
Seeds
Nuts
Coconut milk

SNACKS
Peanuts and raisins
Hummus and Veggies/Organic

NUTRITION GUIDELINES

Blue corn chips
Smoothies
Gluten free Granola

BEVERAGES
Water
Herbal teas
Coconut water
Hemp milk

MISCELLANEOUS
Spirulina Blue Algae
Sea Moss
Yogurt

CHAPTER 13
A PROFESSIONAL WORD ON PROTEIN AND BEETS

"The diesel engine was in fact invented to run on vegetable oil."
- DARYL HANNAH

Protein is the most popular nutrient of all time! It gets more love, conversation, powders and supplements made from it than any other nutrient. The thing is the amount of protein we need is debatable! Its recommend that most people who range from couch potatoes to those who workout about 30 minutes a day 3-5 days a week, need between .8-.9g of protein per kg of body weight a day.

New research has shown that strength training and endurance athlete's protein recommendations range from 1.2 to 1.7g/kg/day. Unfortunately many people in the strength training industry recommend 1 or more grams of protein per pound of body weight a day, which is twice the amount recommended even though evidence shows that the protein consumed above the basic recommendation does not enhance muscle mass/strength gains.

In addition to the amounts of protein needed per day, the timing of when protein is consumed is equally

NUTRITION GUIDELINES

important for optimal results. As little as 20g of high-quality protein, eaten either just before or soon after (within in 2 hours) training may help promote muscle growth.

WHY KILOGRAMS?

To calculate the amount of protein needed, convert the amount of weight in pounds into kilograms. Do that by dividing the weight in pounds by 2.2. For example let's use someone who weighs 150lbs.

150lbs / (2.2) = 68kg

So someone who weighs 150lbs will weigh 68kg. Then to figure out the amount of protein you need, multiply your weight in kg by the recommended ranges we discussed earlier.

68kg x 1.2 – 1.7g of protein = 81-115g of protein a day

So for a person who does strength training and weighs 150lbs they would need a range of 81-115g of protein per day.

POWER PACKED! PUMPKIN SEEDS

Pumpkin seeds are a great source of nutrients for plant-based muscle building.

Here's a list of their nutrients and how they can help build muscle.

Leucine is an amino acid that can help promote fat burning and endurance, and can support increased levels of testosterone.

FAT

Pumpkin seeds are rich in fat. Each 1-oz. serving of pumpkin seeds provides about 14g of fat, which can be beneficial for boosting testosterone.

Zinc and **magnesium** are useful in increasing testosterone levels and sperm count in men. Testosterone is an anabolic hormone that encourages muscle growth.

PROTEIN

Just ¼ cup raw pumpkin seeds has 9.5g of protein, which is useful for rebuilding muscle tissue and fibers.

BEET JUICE AND ENDURANCE

Beet juice can boost stamina. Studies have shown, due to the high concentration of dietary nitrates contained in beets that individuals who drank just 2 cups of beet juice experienced up to a 16 percent increase in endurance compared to those who did not.

NUTRITION GUIDELINES

Through a chain reaction, the body changes nitrates into nitric oxide, which helps with blood flow and blood pressure. The nitrates also reduce the amount of oxygen that is required to produce energy, resulting in a lower overall energy burn for the same amount of muscle power. This reduced energy burn is the reason that endurance is increased by beet juice, since the body is able to perform more work using the same amount of energy as it would without the nitrates. Beets are also high in iron, which help to increase muscle endurance.

If you don't like the taste of beet juice mix it in with other fruits and veggies like apples, carrots and kale.

A few things to consider when drinking beet juice is:

-It may cause your urine or stool to have a red color, which is normal and should not cause concern.

-It may increase your blood sugar levels so those with diabetes or on a sugar restricted diet should either avoid or see how their body responds.

-They are also high in oxalates, which can lead to the development of kidney stones so don't drink it more that 3-4 days a week! Balance is key!

CHAPTER 14
DRINK WATER

"Self-discipline is something like a muscle. The more you exercise it, the stronger it gets.
- DANIEL GOLDSTEIN

Around my way I'm known as the water girl! LOL! Water is REALLY important in general but also if you are weight lifting. The amount of sweating you do, the amount of time and intensity you workout, as well as the types of foods you eat can influence the amount of water you lose and the amount of water that needs to be replaced. As you increase your water intake your body will have to adapt to it and you will have more trips to the bathroom. Increase a little at a time and in about a week or two you should get back to your normal urination routine.

DRINKING WATER HELPS TO:

- Increases Energy and Focus. Just mild dehydration (only 1-2% water loss) can lead to reduced concentration and energy, increased perception of exertion, greater fatigue and negative mood changes.
- Increases Physical Strength. Low-moderate dehydration (about 3% water loss) causes a significant reduction in muscular endurance

NUTRITION GUIDELINES

and power output on weight lifting exercises. Specifically, this means you can do 1-2 fewer reps, or you can lift about 10-20% less weight, with the effects being most profound on lower body lifts. By going into a workout fully hydrated, you are able train more intensely with heavier weights. Increased strength equals greater potential for muscle gains.

- Increases Fat loss. Drinking the right amount of water ensures that your body burns fat for energy. The liver and kidneys work together to burn and get rid of fat. If the body is not properly hydrated the kidneys and liver cannot to their job effectively to burn fat.
- Gets Rid of Toxins. When you are burning fat at a higher rate, there are more toxins than usual due to the increased volume of waste by-products. So proper water intake helps to wash out the toxins.
- Reduced Water Weight Gain. You hold a lot of extra pounds in water weight if you're dehydrated. This is because your body doesn't know when it will get more water, and it must retain the water to keep a balanced water-to-electrolyte ratio. And so, you excrete this excess water weight when you properly hydrate yourself, which decreases the bloated look and help you get shredded.

HOW MUCH WATER SHOULD YOU DRINK?

The traditionally recommended water of eight 8 ounce glasses is a good place to start for people who are not working out but for those doing a lot of physical activity, much more water is needed. Unfortunately, no one-size-fits all amount of water to consume can be recommended but here are a few things to consider.

1. **BODY WEIGHT.**
The more you weigh, the more water you will need. Try using the baseline calculation of (body weight in lbs. ÷ 2 = the number of ounces of water to drink). So someone who weighs 150lbs should drink a minimum of 75oz of water a day (if you have not worked out)

2. **PRE WORKOUT**
Before beginning your workout, water intake should be considered based on the color of your urine (darker indicates improper hydration) several hours ahead of time. If you urine is dark drink 20-30oz 2-3 hours before your workout.

3. **REPLACE WHAT YOU LOSE**.
Replace the fluids you lose from sweating and breathing. It is recommended to frequently drink water during the workout at a rate of about 14oz per hour. After your workout, the goal is to fully replace any fluids.

NUTRITIONAL GUIDELINES

4. DRINK AT A CONTROLLED PACE.
Whatever your actual water intake amount is, it is best to drink it at a relatively consistent pace, rather than drinking large quantities at once. A good way is to decide how much you need a day and divide by 6. Then drink that amount every 1 ½ to 2 hours. You should increase the pace as well as the amount of water you drink before, during, and after strenuous activities and while in hotter environments.

5. DON'T STRESS YOURSELF ABOUT BEING PRECISE.
It's impossible to be truly exact, and it is only necessary to have a "close enough" estimate. If anything, just try out the start with 100oz then work your way up to one gallon per day general recommendation.

Don't O.D. on Water. Yes, it is to possible to overdose on water, although technically, it is a condition called hyponatraemia (water poisoning). It is extremely rare to hear about this happening to people because it requires drinking a whole lot of fluid during a short amount of time. Nonetheless, it can occur and it can be fatal. Practically speaking, though, you should be fine unless you plan on having water-chugging contests with your friends.

6 TIPS TO DRINKING MORE WATER

1. Get a new bottle- Buy a glass or stainless steel bottle with a design and style that fits your lifestyle and helps you to feel motivated.

2. Carry the bottle at all times- Drink during downtimes; while waiting in a bank line, sitting on the train or in traffic, next to your bed at night, etc..

3. Drink morning and night- drink a glass of water (approx. 8oz) when you first wake up and one before bed. That's 2 glasses down!

4. Drink one glass every hour on the hour- If done while at work, when the workday is done your water quota is met.

5. Download an app for your phone or computer- There are apps that will remind you to drink water hourly or you can use the built in alarm settings on your phone!

6. Flavor it- Add various natural twists to your water to enhance the flavor. Ideas include: herbs like mint or small pieces of fruit like berries, cucumber, melons, lemons or limes.

NUTRITION GUIDELINES

COCONUT WATER AND HYDRATION

Coconut water has become very popular lately because it contains carbohydrates and natural electrolytes (sodium and potassium) that help to keep you hydrated. When you exercise three hours or longer in the heat or adverse conditions, your body requires higher levels of simple carbohydrates and electrolytes. Some people choose a sports drink like Gatorade to help refuel the nutrients that were lost. While Sports drinks can help hydrate you many are just artificially colored sugar water with salt and potassium added. Coconut water naturally has carbohydrates, sodium and potassium.

Coconut water does have less sodium than sports drinks so it is recommended to add a pinch of salt or drink 1.5 times more coconut water than the sports drink to get the same nutrients.

COCONUT WATER VS SPORTS DRINKS
Ounce per ounce, most unflavored coconut water contains

5.45 calories, 1.3g sugar, 61 milligrams (mg) of potassium, and 5.45mg of sodium compared to Gatorade, which has 6.25 calories, 1.75g of sugar, 3.75mg of potassium, and 13.75mg of sodium.

CHAPTER 15
REST AND RECOVERY

"Sleep is the best meditation."
- DALAI LAMA

Another thing besides water intake that I emphasized with Khnum was getting enough rest. He is so busy with music, writing, business and the other 1 million ideas that he has on a dally basis that sleep can easily become a side note for him. Sleep in general is important to build your immune system. I like to think of sleep similarly to charging my phone or computer. If you don't charge it you can't use it! When you are sleep your immune system recharges and also uses that time to help to heal and repair parts of the body and keep you healthy. Studies show that a minimum of 8 hours of sleep is best for optimal health and muscle growth.

THE IMPORTANCE OF SLEEP AND MUSCLE BUILDING

1. Growth Hormones- your body releases a growth hormone while you're at rest during the night. Since growth hormones are closely correlated to muscle-size increases, you want to maximize this hormone as much as you can. In women, the growth hormone is released in smaller bursts throughout the day. In men, however, there tends to be a single burst released,

NUTRITION GUIDELINES

and it is heavily correlated with the onset of sleep, specifically deep sleep. Guys who sleep less and spend less time in deep sleep tend to notice a decline in the overall growth hormone released, and this slows down the rate of muscle building.

2. Cortisol- cortisol is a hormone that directly opposes muscle building and encourages the breakdown of body tissue. If you don't get enough rest cortisol levels of the body are increased and will take you further from the optimum recovery state that you want to be in before your next workout.

3. Muscle Repair- Every time you lift weights in the gym and overload your muscles, tiny micro-tears in the muscle tissues are created. These tears are repaired and built back up when you are sleep. When your body is repaired you notice strength and size gains.

4. Metabolism - Metabolism converts the fuel in the food we eat into the energy needed to power everything we do, from moving to thinking to growing. Sleep helps to regulate our metabolism and keep it working properly. If your metabolism is functioning properly you body will burn fat while retaining lean muscle. Also a lack of sleep tends to suppress the thyroid hormone, which is the primary regulator of how many calories you burn on a daily basis. If you want to burn off fat as best as possible, it's important that you maximize your metabolism.

SIGNS THAT YOU ARE NOT GETTING ENOUGH REST:

If you can't recover properly between sessions, your body will give you signals. These signals can be different from person to person, but you will stall and get stuck if you ignore it and keep pushing.

SOME OF THESE SIGNS INCLUDE:

1. Can't/don't want to eat as much because you are tired
2. Feeling lethargic or fatigued
3. Can't focus as well
4. Having a harder time falling asleep
5. Random pains in the joints/tendons/ligaments

Sleep is said to be the cousin of death and that may very well be true metaphorically but when it comes to health and fitness sleep is the cousin of Life.

NUTRITION GUIDELINES

CHAPTER 16
LOOSING TO GAIN: A RECIPE FOR SUCCESS

"Focused, hard work is the real key to success. Keep your eyes on the goal, and just keep taking the next step towards completing it. If you aren't sure which way to do something, do it both ways and see what works better."
- JOHN CARMACK

Overall we saw that the Lean Bulk Phase was the most effective for Stic to gain weight with the least amount of fat and for him to follow his eating plan and be satisfied with his meals.

The lean bulk phase was a good balance between the bulk and cut phase for Stic. He did not feel as constricted by the diet and it was easier for him to follow. He was able to still gain muscle, lose fat and get shredded. We calculated his nutrient needs and focused on mostly whole foods that were low in fat and he ate 3 meals and 2-3 snacks a day. We made sure he was getting in a minimum of 100oz of water a day and getting 7-8 hours of sleep most nights.

NUTRITION GUIDELINES

NUTRITION TAKEAWAYS

As you can see nutrition plays a major role in building muscle. What you eat and drink becomes the fuel for your workouts and the building blocks of your muscles. Focusing on your macro nutrient intake, calories and meal timing will have a huge impact on your results. This experiment was really important because we actually showed that it is possible to gain weight on a plant based diet and with out added supplements. Plant based or not it takes a lot of discipline to reach your fitness goals and I salute those who put in that work!

The process of building muscle and gaining weight can seem overwhelming so here are a few basic tips to keep in mind when gaining plant based muscle.

START WITH WHOLE FOODS

Focusing on whole foods (beans, nuts/seeds, fruits, vegetables and whole grains) is a good place to start. Whole foods are easy fuel for your body to process and will not turn into fat as quickly as processed foods. Also a variety of balanced nutrients from whole foods makes sure you are getting the adequate amount of vitamins and minerals needed for muscle growth, energy and maintaining the immune system.

REDUCE PROCESSED FOODS

Most processed foods come in the form of carbohydrates. Carbohydrates are important because they are stored in your muscles as glycogen and along with protein help keep your muscles full and large and fuel them during workouts. Instead of eating the processed forms of carbs like bread and desserts, for most meals, stick with slow-digesting carb sources such as whole grains, oatmeal, sweet potatoes, beans, fruit and vegetables.

DRINK UP

Hydration falls right after diet and exercise when it comes to gaining muscle. Start with half your body weight in ounces daily and increase amounts when you work out.

GET IN GREENS

Green vegetables are a great source of calcium for the plant based lifestyles. Calcium is a mineral used in the contraction of muscles, as well as in the maintenance of bones. Attempt to include greens in 4 out of your 6 meals a day. Add them in fresh juices, smoothies and as a side or a snack.

NUTRITION GUIDELINES

EAT UP

A basic rule of thumb is to eat 3 meals and 2-3 snacks a day. Eat a meal that contains quality protein and carbs every 2-3 hours to ensure a steady supply of energy and amino acids for muscle growth all day long, helping you gain mass and stay lean. The key is to keep every meal approximately the same size. Do not gorge out at any one meal. Be disciplined enough to eat smaller meals or else your body will begin to store extra calories as fat.

WHEN IN DOUBT EAT PROTEIN

When its time to eat again and you are not sure what to grab, choose a high protein food like, Tempeh, tofu, quinoa or nuts/seeds. This will help to keep your muscles growing and to keep you feeling full and satisfied.

GET SOME ZZZZ'S

Get a minimum of 7-8 hours of sleep at night to help the body to build and repair the effects of muscle training. Sleep also helps to keep your immunity strong and keeps you focused and energized for your workouts!

STAY CONSISTENT

Consistency with your food intake is important. I've heard some people say they get tired of chewing or bored with eating the same foods. If you are tired of chewing substitute some meals for smoothies and if you are tired of the same foods find new recipes to add to your food choices.

PLAN YOUR MEALS

Planning your meals helps you to stay on track with your program and reduces the guessing game of what you should eat. That may sound a little boring but when you are hungry after a workout and have not planned your meals out it will be easier for you to slip up and choose something that's not part of your program and hinder your results.

NUTRITION GUIDELINES

LEAN BULK RECIPES

CHAMPION CHICKPEAS & KALE

1 bunch kale
1 can chickpeas
2 Tsp garlic
¼ Cup low sodium vegetable broth

Directions:
1. Heat a medium cast iron or non stick on medium heat. Add oil and chickpeas into the pan.
2. Lay flat and cook for about 5 minutes browning lightly.
3. Add all ingredients except veggie broth sauté for two minutes. Then add broth cook 5 more minutes or until kale is at desired consistency.

Makes 2 servings
Amount of nutrients per serving
Calories 255
Fat 4g
Protein 15g
Carbs 47g

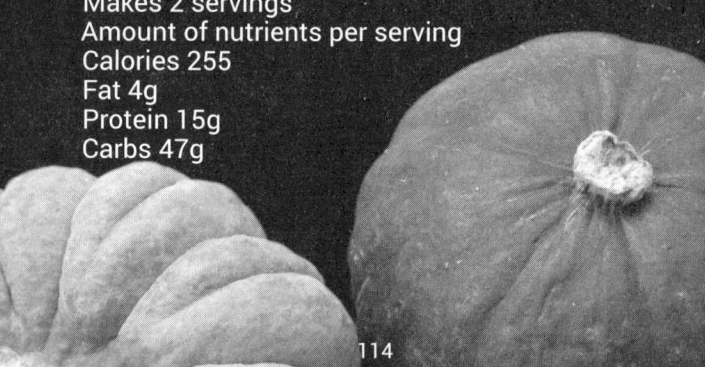

IRON SHIRT PAN FRIED TOFU

Ingredients:

1 Block tofu
¼ Cup veggie broth or water
1 Tsp garlic powder
¼ Tsp salt
1 Tsp chili powder

Directions:
1. Cut the tofu in steaks
2. Add reaming ingredients to a flat dish and mix well.
3. Add the tofu and marinate for at least 30 minutes.
4. Heat a nonstick or cast iron pan on med high heat. Add tofu and the oil at the same time.
5. Brown on both sides.
6. Add marinade cover and simmer 10 minutes checking to make sure all the liquid has not left.

Makes 2 servings
Amount of nutrients per serving
Calories 123
Fat 7g
Protein 14g
Carbs 5g

NUTRITION GUIDELINES

SIDEWALK CRACKING SCRAMBLED KALE & TOFU

Ingredients:

2 Tablespoons oil
1 Extra firm block tofu
3 Cups shredded kale
1 Teaspoon smoked paprika
½ Cup onions
1 Tablespoon minced garlic
1 ¼ Teaspoon sea salt or to taste
2 Teaspoons granulated garlic or garlic powder
¼ Cup low sodium vegetable broth

Directions:
1. Heat a medium cast iron or nonstick on medium heat.
   Add oil and crumble tofu into the pan.
2. Lay flat and cook for about 5 minutes browning lightly. Then flip over lay flat and cook for 5 more minutes.
3. Add all ingredients except veggie broth sauté for two minutes. Then add broth cook 5 more minutes or until kale is at desired consistency.

Makes 2 servings
Amount of nutrients per serving

Calories 323
Fat 17g
Protein 28g
Carbs 25g

***Kale can be substituted for broccoli, chard or spinach

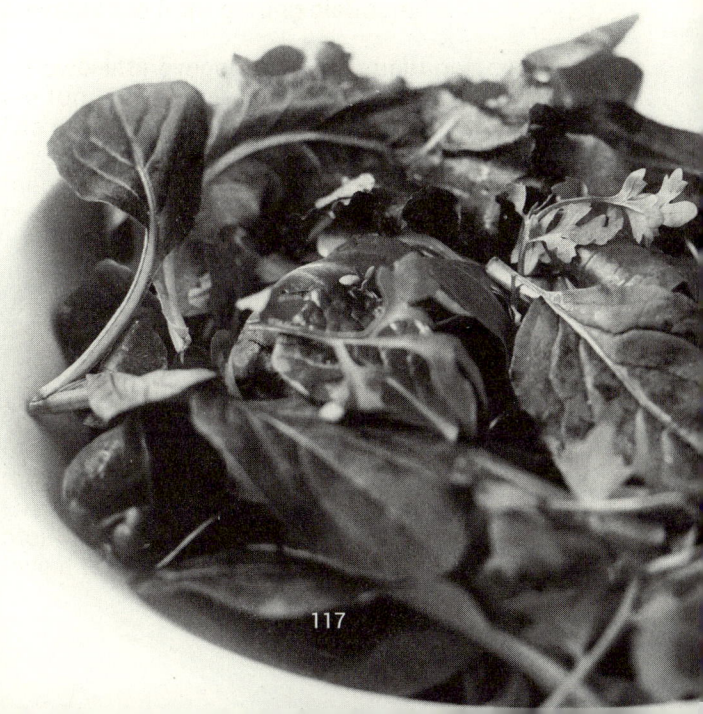

NUTRITIONAL GUIDELINES

POWER HOUSE PORTOBELLO MUSHROOMS

Ingredients:
4 large whole portabella mushrooms
½ Block hemp tofu, divided
¼ Cup tomato sauce divided
1 Cup Organic Baby Spinach, divided
1 Tsp Italian seasoning divided
½ Tsp granulated garlic
Dash of salt

Directions:
1. Preheat oven to 400.
2. Remove stems from mushrooms and rub tops with damp towel until clean.
3. Lay mushrooms on a baking sheet.
4. Starting with 1 mushroom, spread 1 Tblsp of tomato sauce on inside, sprinkle ¼ Tsp of Italian seasoning, a dash of salt and granulated garlic.
5. ¼ Cup spinach and 1/4 cup tofu
6. Repeat for other three mushrooms.
7. Bake for 20-25 minutes

2 mushrooms are 1 serving
Amount of nutrients per serving
Calories 152
Fat 6g
Protein 14g
Carbs 16g

IRON SPLIT PEA SOUP

Ingredients:
1 Cup yellow split peas
8 Cups water
1/3 Cup chopped tomatoes
2 Tsp minced garlic
2 Tsp fresh ginger grated
1 Tsp ground coriander
The juice of 1 lemon
1/2 Tsp sea salt

Directions:
1. Bring water to a boil and add split peas.
2. Cook uncovered on med/high for 1 hour, stirring occasionally to prevent sticking. Soup should be thin so add more water if needed.
3. Add veggies and spices except salt and cook for 30 more min. Stir occasionally
4. Turn soup off and add lemon juice and salt.

Makes 5 servings
Amount of nutrients per serving
Calories 96
Fat 0g
Protein 8g
Carbs 24g

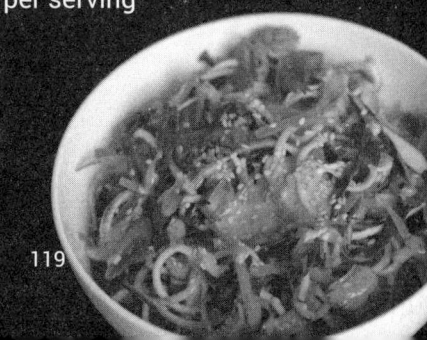

NUTRITION GUIDELINES

GOOD MORNING SALUTE

1 large apple
½ Cup peanuts or almonds
2 Tblsp raisins
Pinch of cinnamon
Pinch of lemon juice

Directions:
1. Combine all ingredients into a food processor ad mix well

Makes 1 serving

Amount of nutrients per serving
Calories 552
Fat 37g
Protein 18g
Carbs 49g

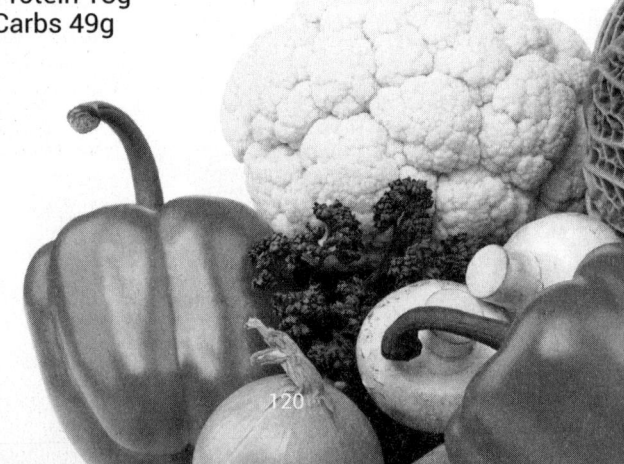

HERCULEAVES SNACK SMOOTHIE

Ingredients:
1 cup Collard Greens or kale
1 banana
1 tsp Spirulina Powder
3 tbsp Pumpkin Seeds
1 ½ cups Hemp Milk

Directions:
1. All ingredients to nutri bullet or high powered blender and mix well

Makes 1 serving
Calories 461
Fat 30g
Protein 20g
Carbs 34g

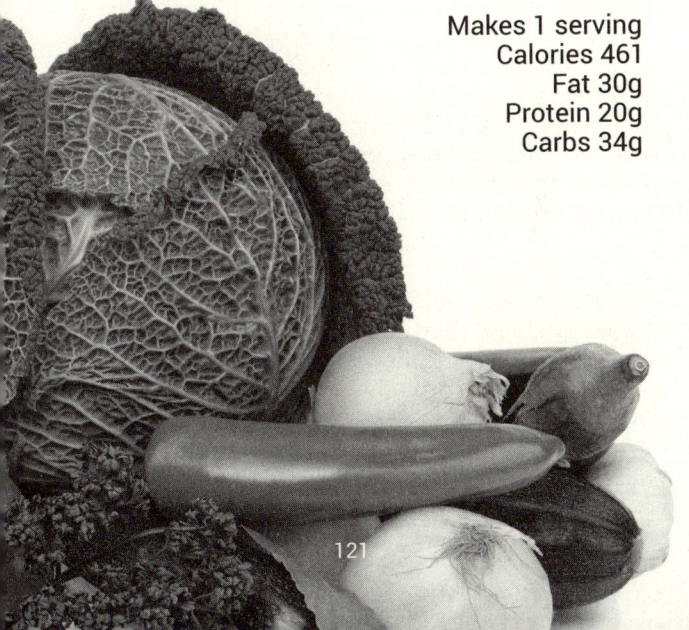

NUTRITION GUIDELINES

HULK MILK GREEN SMOOTHIE

Ingredients:
1 Cup Swiss chard
1/3 cucumber with peel
1 Tsp ginger root about ½ inch
1 gala apple
1 ½ Cup water
1 Tsp Spirulina

Directions;
1. All ingredients to nutri bullet or high powered blender and mix well

Makes 1 serving
Amount of nutrients per serving
Calories 101
Fat 0g
Protein 3g
Carbs 20g

PLANT BEAST
PRE/POST WORKOUT SMOOTHIE

Ingredients:
1 Cup hemp milk
1 banana
1/2 Cup blueberries or strawberries
3 tablespoons peanut butter
1 Tsp Spirulina
1 Cup water
1 Tsp ginger root
1 Tblsp soaked chia seeds

Directions:
1. Mix well in high powered blender or nutri bullet

Makes 1 serving

Amount of nutrients per serving
Calories 644
Fat 30g
Protein 19g
Carbs 75g

NUTRITIONAL GUIDELINES

GLADIATOR THAI FRIED QUINOA

Ingredients:
3 Cups cold cooked quinoa preferably a day old (1 Cup dry equals 3 Cups cooked)

Sauce:
1 Tablespoon + 1 Teaspoon Thai red curry paste
2 Teaspoons toasted sesame oil
2 Tablespoons water
1 ¼ Teaspoon sea salt
½ Teaspoon chili garlic sauce (optional depending on how spicy you like it)

Veggies:
1 tablespoon oil
1 ¼ Cup small onion, diced
¼ Cup small bell pepper, diced
1 Teaspoon minced garlic
1 Cup frozen mixed veggies

Garnish:
Lightly chopped cilantro, mint or Thai basil for garnish
2 Tablespoons roasted crushed peanuts (optional)

Directions:
1. In a small bowl, whisk the sauce ingredients

together until they form a paste. Set aside.
2. Heat oil in a wok. Add onion and sauté until translucent. Then add the garlic, mixed veggies and bell pepper, and sauté for about 3 minutes.
3. Add the sauce and stir on high heat for about 30 seconds.
4. Add the cooked quinoa to the wok. Using a wide spatula, gently and quickly stir the quinoa to incorporate everything. Stir fry for about 2-3 minutes.
5. Top with crushed peanuts, chopped cilantro, mint or Thai basil.

Makes 4 servings
Amount of nutrients per serving
Calories 172
Fat 8g
Protein 4g
Carbs 21g

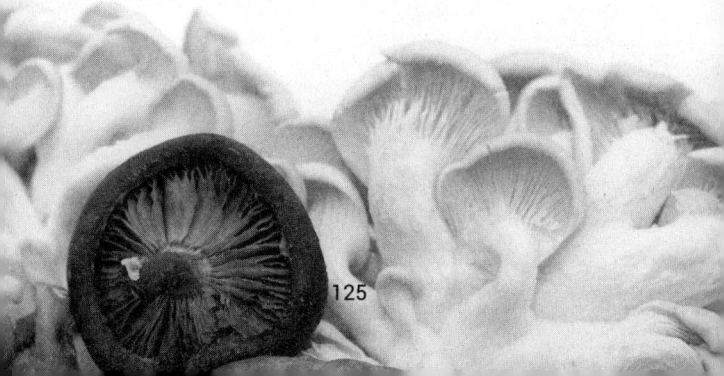

NUTRITION GUIDELINES

GANGSTA LEAN GARLIC GREEN BEANS

Ingredients:

1 lb green beans
½ Cup low sodium vegetable broth
3 Tsp minced garlic
1/4 Tsp sea salt

Directions:
1. Blanch green beans in a large pot of boiling water for 2 minute and remove
2. Add vegetable broth and garlic to pan and sauté on medium for 3 minutes
3. Add green beans and Stir fry for 5 min on med high constantly mixing so garlic does not burn
4. Turn heat off cover for 3 min add ¼ Cup water if necessary.

Makes 3 servings
Amount of nutrients per serving
Calories 57
Fat 0g
Protein 3g
Carbs 12g

LEAF UP SAUTÉED GREENS (BROCCOLI OR KALE)

Ingredients
2 Cups broccoli or kale
½ Cup Portobello mushroom
¼ Cup low sodium vegetable broth
2 Tsp minced garlic
½ Tsp sea salt

Directions
1. Chop veggies.
2. Add garlic and veggie broth to a pan on medium heat. Sauté for 2 minutes
3. Add remaining ingredients cover and reduce heat to med/low for 5 minutes.
4. Add more water if necessary remove cover and sauté 2 more minutes.

Makes 2 servings
Amount of nutrients per serving
Calories 43
Fat 0g
Protein 3g
Carbs 8g

NUTRITION GUIDELINES

RON ENDURANCE BEET SALAD

Ingredients:
2 Cups beets, cut in small cubes
½ Cup onion, minced
½ Jalapeño, seeded and minced
2 Tablespoons olive oil
Juice of 1 lemon
½ Teaspoon sea salt or to taste

Directions:
1. Soak beets in water for 5 minutes then peel with a vegetable peeler.
2. Cut beets into small cubes and boil in a medium pot for 20 minutes or until soft.
3. In a medium boil mix the remaining ingredients.
4. Strain beets then add to bowl.
5. Toss ingredients. Serve warm or cold.

Makes 4 servings

Amount of nutrients per serving

Calories 67
Fat 4 g
Protein 1g
Carbs 9g

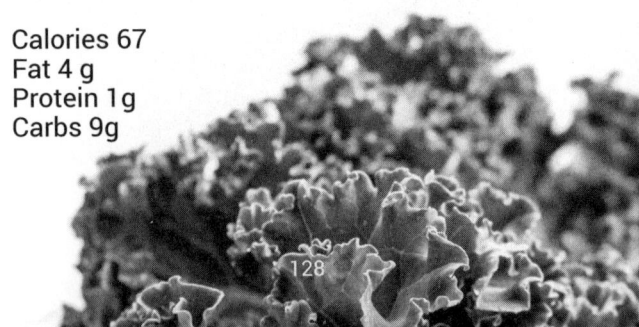

IRON MAN KALE SALAD

Ingredients:
5 Cups (about 1lb) Raw Kale
2 Tblsp Nutritional Yeast
½ Cup Sun dried Tomatoes
1 tablespoon Sesame oil
1 Cup warm Water
1 Cup Pacific Foods low sodium Vegetable Broth
1/4 Tsp Sea Salt
1 Tsp Garlic powder
Juice of ½ lemon

Directions:
1. Soak tomatoes in warm water and let sit for 20 minutes until soft.
2. Cut kale in thin strips and wash.
3. Mix oils, spices, vegetable broth and lemon juice in a medium bowl.
4. Cut tomatoes into this strips or pieces. Add tomatoes and soaking water to oil mixture.
5. Add a little kale at a time to mixture and massage until kale turns limp about 2 minutes.

Makes 4 servings
Amount of nutrients per serving
Calories 103
Fat 4g
Protein 4g
Carbs 15g

NUTRITION GUIDELINES

BIG & LEAFY GREEN SALAD WITH AVOCADO

Ingredients:
1 head of green leaf lettuce
1 cucumber
1 Cup radishes
1 Cup cherry tomatoes
½ Cup shredded raw beets
1 avocado

Directions:
1. Cut all ingredients in bite size pieces toss well.

Makes 3 servings

Amount of nutrients per serving
Calories 165
Fat 10g
Protein 5g
Carbs 18g

TRIUMPHANT CHIA SEEDS

1 Tblsp chia seeds
1 Cup water

Add ingredients to a glass or ceramic container and store in the refrigerator and use for smoothies or on top of oatmeal.

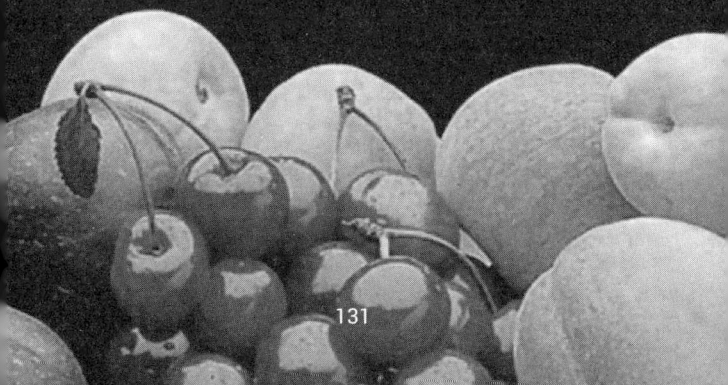

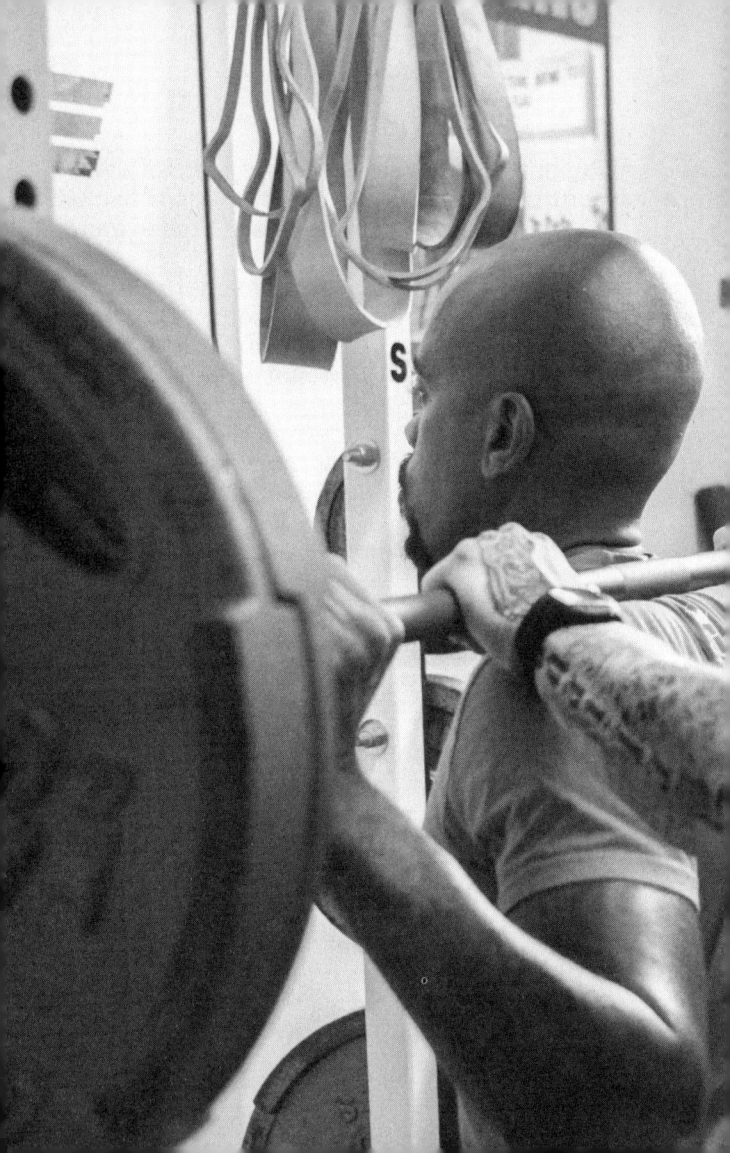

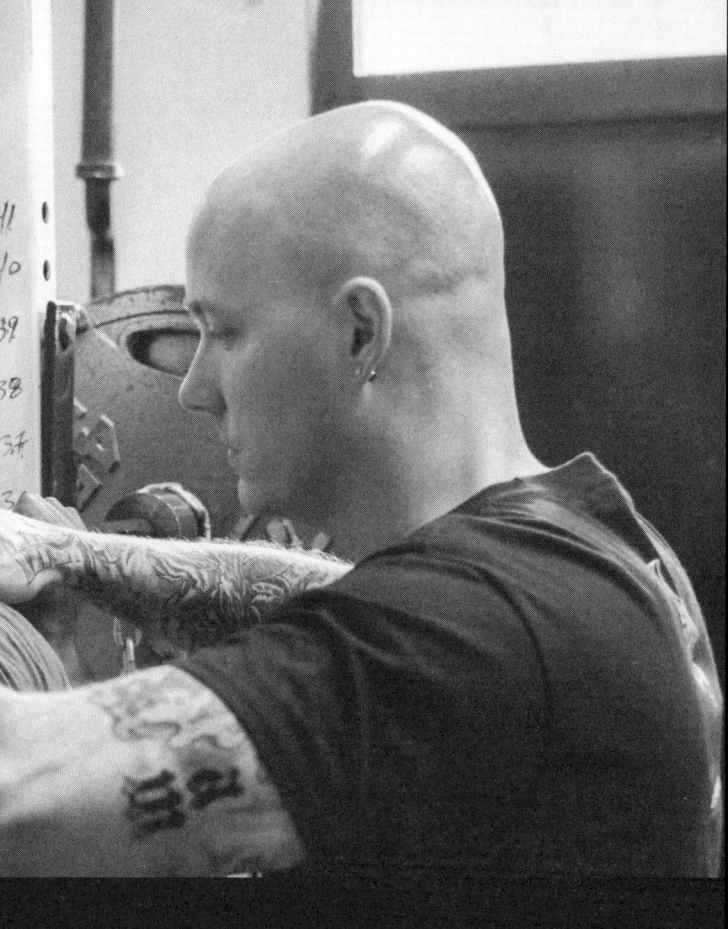

SECTION 3: SCOTT SHETLER NSCA-CPT
THE TRAINING: IRON SHARPENS MAN

THE TRAINING: IRON SHARPENS MAN

CHAPTER 17
THE MAN WITH THE VEGAN IRON FISTS

"Strength does not come from physical capacity.
It comes from an indomitable will."
- MAHATMA GANDHI

I met Stic through a project I did as a benefit for the animal welfare organization, Mercy For Animals. One of my purposes in life is to give back and support organizations engaged in animal rights and welfare, so I authored a book titled, "Plant-Based Performance: A Compassionate Approach to Health and Fitness", along with the help of 18 other plant-based athletes, health and fitness professionals, and enthusiasts. After learning that Stic followed a plant-based diet I asked him to be part of this project. After submitting his section of the book, we met at my training center where he proposed the idea for a joint project, which eventually became this book.

He had been struggling to gain muscular weight, and as a long distance runner with a naturally thin frame this became more of a challenge. His goal was to add 20 lbs of muscle while continuing to follow his passion of distance running. In addition he wanted to do this all while following a plant-based (vegan) diet without the aid of supplements, so no powders or pills of any kind,

THE TRAINING: IRON SHARPENS MAN

and he wanted to accomplish this goal in a 4-month time frame.

One of Stic's mottos is "teamwork make the dream work" and knowing that this goal would be difficult to accomplish on his own, he enlisted me as his strength and conditioning trainer, and his wife Afya, a plant-based holistic nutrition specialist, to ensure his training and nutrition was where it needed to be to accomplish his goal.

This made his goal twofold. Not only did he want the personal accomplishment, he also wanted to be an inspiration to other "hard-gainers", or naturally thin individuals who have a hard time putting on weight, and as a result our "Eat Plants, Lift Iron" movement was born!

A SIFU OF STRENGTH

In this section of the book I will provide information on strength training to help give you an understanding of the science behind training and program design as well as provide specific information on the training, and individual training blocks, we did for Stic's transformation. I will also share some various tips such as my top recommended exercises for strength and muscle gain.

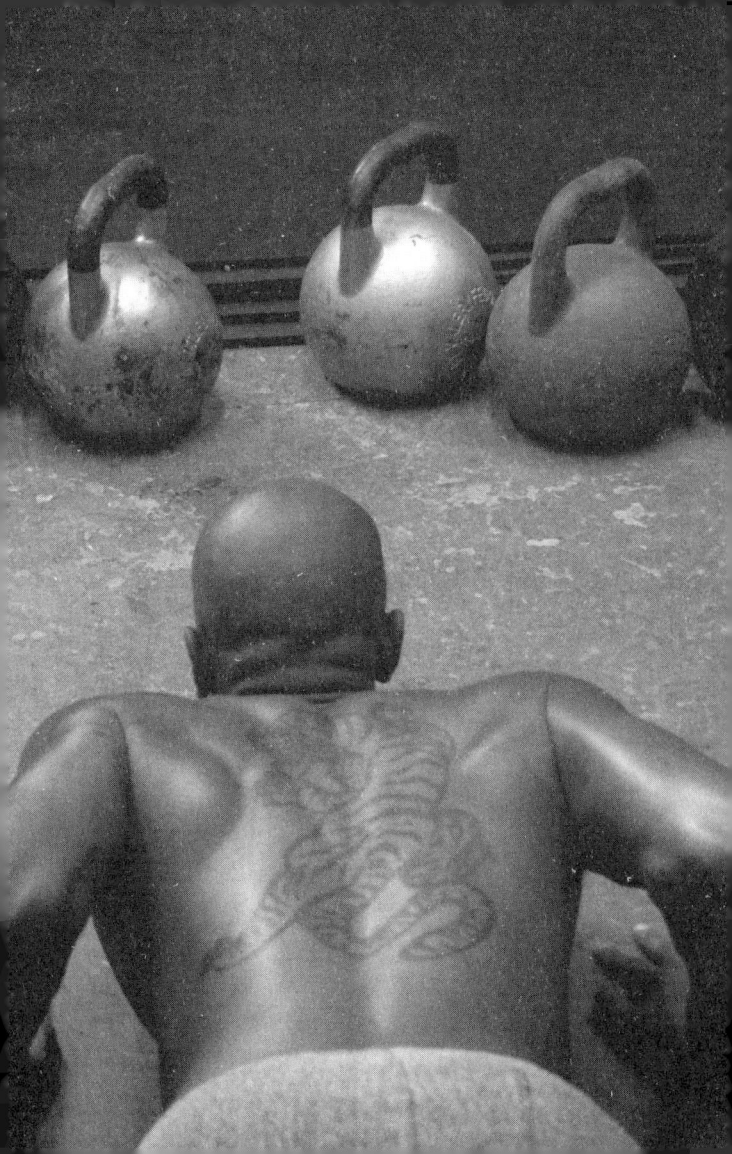

THE TRAINING: IRON SHARPENS MAN

It is my hope that after you read this section of the book not only will you be inspired by the work Stic and I did together, but have enough of an understanding of these basic principles to apply to your training to help you get the most out of the time you spend in the gym.

Let's get to it!

STRENGTH TRAINING TERMS AND DEFINITIONS

Before we get to the nuts and bolts of the program, I need to present some terms and definitions that will help you better understand the details of the programming as it comes up in the book. Some of these terms you may be familiar with, some you may not. These are just intended to help you make sense of the details in Stic's training plan.

- Sets A set is a group of repetitions performed in succession, i.e. "A set of ten reps."
- Repetitions or "Reps" A repetition is one complete lift from start to finish.
- Intensity. Intensity refers to the amount of weight used for a lift, usually expressed as a percentage of a 1-repetition maximum.
- Volume. Volume is the amount of work done in a given workout. The sum total of the number of sets, repetitions, and weight used for a workout is the volume of that specific

session.
- Hypertrophy Building muscle mass.
- Anabolic Building up
- Catabolic Breaking down

THE SCIENCE OF STRENGTH TRAINING

When I talk about the science of strength training I am referring to set principles that yield a specific result. I differ from some in the field of exercise science in that I do not need a peer-reviewed study to validate methods. My work is done in the gym, and networking with other professionals who get similar results. If I see a trend that works, I do not wait for science to validate it. This is not meant to discredit the scientific method at all, but I rely both on science as well as empirical evidence when building my training programs.

I think that one of the most important factors to understand when we talk about the science of training is the recommended repetitions for the exercises. In Stic's sample training logs you will see some exercises done for sets of low reps and some for sets of higher reps. This will help you understand how repetition prescriptions apply to the training goal. Keep in mind that it is imperative to use a weight that only allows you to hit the target repetition range in order to achieve the desired training effect. For instance, if I recommend a set of bench presses for 4-6 reps and you use a weight you could get 10-12 reps with, you will not achieve the

THE TRAINING: IRON SHARPENS MAN

desired training effect of that set.
- 1-5 repetitions - optimal for developing maximal strength.
- 6-12 repetitions - optimal for hypertrophy (building muscle).
- 12-20+ repetitions - optimal for developing muscular endurance.

As a general rule of thumb for managing the training volume, the lower the reps - the higher the sets and the higher the reps the lower the sets. When you are working on maximal strength, performing more sets in the 1-5 rep range is ideal.

STRENGTH AND THE CENTRAL NERVOUS SYSTEM

The use of very heavy weights, i.e. 90% or greater of the 1 rep max, requires a greater response from the central nervous system (CNS) then training with lighter weights for higher reps.

The development of strength is more of a by-product of training the CNS than the muscular system. With this being the case, an approach that utilizes heavy weights, for multiple sets of low reps generally provides the greatest training effect. While the development of strength is largely neural, muscle mass does play a role, albeit when the nervous system has been properly stimulated with the appropriate loads.

When we lift maximal and near-maximal weights, the CNS works hard to contract as much of the available muscle fiber in the working muscles as possible. Over time the CNS becomes more conditioned and efficient to this task and as a result the muscles fire in a more coordinated effort, thus resulting in a greater level of strength.

When you are stronger, you can use heavier weights for the higher volume work that accompanies a mass building training phase. This will allow you to continue to build muscle at a fast rate by preventing the body from adapting to the training load.

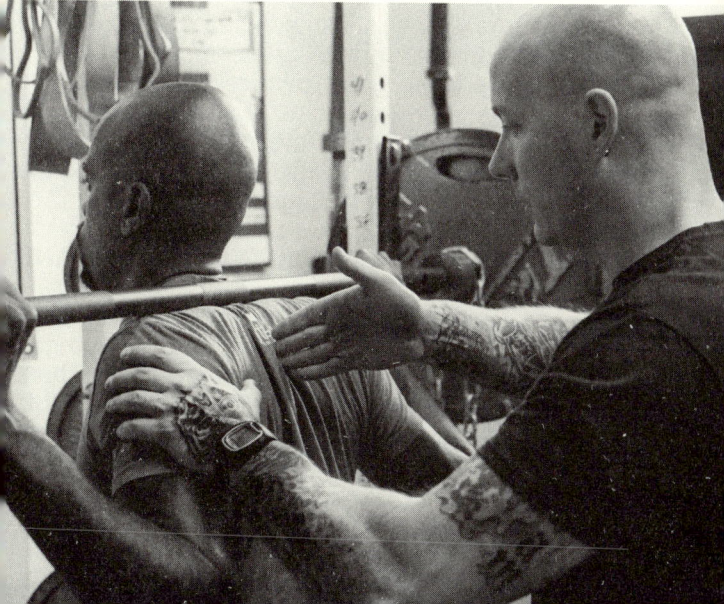

THE TRAINING: IRON SHARPENS MAN

If your goal is muscle endurance, performing fewer sets (1-3) of higher reps (12-20 or more) will provide the best result. If muscle size is the goal the recommendation falls right between maximal strength and maximal endurance.

However, even though performing sets with weights that allow for 6-12 reps is optimal for building muscle mass, I feel it is very important to train with heavier weights some of the time, as strength and muscle go hand in hand.

FACTORS FOR DEVELOPING THE TRAINING PLAN

Many factors come into play when setting up the training plan and deciding on the training volume, such as training experience, goals, injuries, etc.. This makes the development of training a highly individualized process. The above is simply meant to give you a very general idea, and help you make some sense of the sample training plans we provide in this book.

BEING A GOOD TRAINER IS BOTH A SCIENCE AND AN ART.

We are providing sample workouts so that you can get an idea of how Stic's training program was built and progressed through each phase. The sample programs are excerpts from his actual training log. We did not want to "prescribe" the exact program for you, the reader, to follow, as your goals may not be what Stic was trying to accomplish. Rather we hope that the sample programs will provide some inspiration for you to evaluate your training plan and make any changes to it that may benefit your personal goals. If you would like a program developed specifically for you and your goals, both Afya and I offer consultation services in our areas of expertise, and our contact info is located in the back of the book in the About the Authors section.

THE TRAINING: IRON SHARPENS MAN

CHAPTER 18
AIMING FOR THE GOAL

" Our goals can only be reached through a vehicle of a plan, in which we must fervently believe, and upon which we must vigorously act. There is no other route to success."
- PABLO PICASSO

When building a program it is essential that a clearly defined goal be considered. As we've stated numerous times in this book, Stic's goal was pretty cut and dry.

Gain 20 lbs. of mass in four months while still keeping up with long distance running and following a whole-food, plant-based diet, without the aid of supplements.

Perfect. Now that the goal is established it is easy to dictate the training and nutrition.

THE ASSESSMENT

Once we had a goal in place it was time to do an assessment to see where Stic was at in relation to where he wanted to go with his goal.

THE TRAINING: IRON SHARPENS MAN

The assessment is a crucial part of the preparation process as it allows me to find out everything I need to know about my clients physically, any injuries or other issues that may be affected by training, training experience, and other information that will determine the way I set up the training plan. It also allows me to look at my clients structurally to see if there are any glaring muscular imbalances that need addressing.

Since Stic's goal had to do with adding mass, and eventually decreasing body-fat, I also had to monitor his body composition using his scale weight and a body-fat analysis we conducted using skin fold measurements.

After testing his body composition what we found was that Stic was a tall lean guy with a typical runner's build, was walking around at 6'2", 168 lbs. and his body-fat was at a low 9.42%.

WEAK SPOTS

I determined that one of the reasons he was not carrying the amount of muscle he wanted was due to his training. His current training plan was more conditioning-based and lacked the multiple-joint, compound lifts that are essential for build both muscle size and strength. Lifts like the squat, bench press, and dead lift have been used successfully by many athletes when increased size and strength is the goal. He was training more like an old school boxer, on a steady diet of running, calisthenics, and lighter weight exercises.

After this assessment I knew not only could we accomplish his goal of a 20 lb. gain very easily, I was also sure that it wouldn't take the entire 4 months. Even with the running, I expected that once he began training the big lifts hard, and eating a ton of calories, he was going to blow up.

DEVELOPING THE STRATEGIC APPROACH

With the assessment out the way I began building the training plan. In addition to tracking his body composition, I wanted to use some of the basic strength movements as "indicator lifts". This would allow me to see the progress in strength over the course of our training program.

I selected the squat, bench press, and trap bar (hex bar) dead lift as the lifts I would monitor. To begin I needed to determine the 1 rep max (or estimated 1 rep max) of each of these lifts so that I had a baseline to monitor his progress with.

I spent the first 3 weeks introducing the movements and working on technique, as I acclimated him to this type of training, then we took 1 rep max attempts in each of these movements.

THE TRAINING: IRON SHARPENS MAN

I will detail in specifics his pre-and post-goal body composition assessments, as well as detail the progress in his indicator lifts in a reference table later in this section.

FEEDING THE FOCUS

Stic's nutrition was to be handled by Afya. She and I consulted on some basic things like body composition, calorie requirements, and nutrient timing to make sure that his diet worked synergistically with the training allowing him not only enough fuel to train, but most importantly a surplus of calories to assist in the muscle building process.

CHAPTER 19
THE REGIMEN

"Excellence is a Habit."
- ARISTOTLE

I decided to divide the training into specific blocks, each with it's own goal. After meeting with Stic I decided that a 3-day per week training split would be optimal as it would allow us to do the strength training work necessary to accomplish his goal and still allow time for him to get 2-3 distance runs in per week, all while providing enough recovery time for the body to repair and grow post-training. Essentially we would be hitting each muscle group hard, 1-2 times per week. This would stimulate the body to grow, then by refuelling with healthy nutrition and resting adequately, the muscle growth would occur.

TRAINING BLOCK 1 ASSESSMENTS, ACCLIMATION AND TECHNIQUE

Duration: 3-4 weeks

Objective: Introduce training plan, establish technique for the indicator lifts, determine 1 repetition maximum for indicator lifts

THE TRAINING: IRON SHARPENS MAN

The initial training block was an introductory phase that was to be 3-4 weeks. The primary focus of this training block was to introduce the indicator lifts and accessory exercises. The goal of the accessory exercises are to support the indicator lifts, balance out the program, and address specific weak points. This is the phase in which I wanted to gradually raise the training volume so that he had the necessary base to move on to a higher volume phase in block 2.

The indicator lifts were trained in a low repetition range to allow for heavier loads to be used. Typically the set and repetition range was 3 sets x 3-5 reps. We often follow this with a back off set or two of a lighter weight and higher repetitions to help increase the overall training volume for the purpose of building muscle mass.

The accessory exercises were typically done in a higher repetition range with moderate, to moderately heavy weights; just enough to hit the target rep range. A typical set and rep range for an accessory lift would be 3-4 sets x 8-12 reps.

This training block ended after working up to 1 repetition maximums in the indicator lifts.

SAMPLE TRAINING WEEK FROM BLOCK 1

*Note - training plan is written as "weight" x "reps" / "sets"

Monday, 10/28/13 - bench press and upper body accessory warm up with Indian clubs and suspended push up and rows

*chins: 3-5 reps w/ every set of bench press

1. Bench press: warm-up sets - barx15, 65x10, 80x8, 95x5; work sets - 115x3 / 3 sets; back-off sets - 95x8, 95x7, 85x8

2a. Incline dumbbell bench press: 30x8; 25x8,6

2b. Seated row: 70x12,10,8

3a. Dumbbell skull crusher: 15x10-12 / 3

3b. Barbell curl: 45x10-12 / 3

4a. Lateral raise: 10x10-15 / 3

4b. Ab wheel: bwx10-15 / 3

Wednesday, 10/30/13 - squat, trap bar dead lift, and lower body accessory warm-up: body weight squats x 10-15; kettle bell swings 16kg x 15 / 3

1. Squat: warm-up sets - barx10, 65x8, 95x5; work sets - 115x5, 135x5, 155x5;

back-off sets - 115x10, 95x15

2. Trap-bar dead lift: warm-up sets - 135x5, 155x5; work sets - 185x3, 205x3, 225x3; back-off sets - 185x5 / 2

3a. Split squat: 10x10 / 3

3b. Glute/hamstring raise (GHR): bwx10,8,6

4a. Calf raise: 35x20-25 / 3

THE TRAINING: IRON SHARPENS MAN

4b. GHR sit-up: bwx20-25 / 3
5. Kettle bell snatch: 12kgx10,8,6

Friday, 11/1/13 - upper body accessory
Warm up with Indian clubs and suspended push up and rows
 *chins: 3-5 reps w/ every set of press
1. Overhead press: barx10, 65x8 / 2, 65x6 / 2
2a. Close-grip bench press: 85x10 / 4
2b. Lat pulldown: 70x12 / 4
3a. "Ez bar" skull crusher: 40x10-15 / 4
3b. Dumbbell curl: 20x10-15 / 4
4a. Bent over lateral: 15x12-15 / 3
4b. Leg raises: bwx20-25 / 3

TRAINING BLOCK 2: BULKING PHASE

Duration: 6 weeks

Objective: dramatically increase volume, rapid development of muscle mass

For training block 2 we implemented an approach called the 10 sets method. I first learned of this program through the work of world-class strength coach, Charles Poliquin, in a program he presented known as German Volume Training, or GVT.

This is a great method for quickly developing muscle mass. In a nutshell you select one exercise for each body-part and perform 10 sets of 10 repetitions with approximately 60-90 seconds of rest between each set. You should begin this plan using about 60% of your 1 repetition maximum for each exercise and increase the weight when you are able to get all 10 sets of 10 reps.

According to Poliquin this program works by attacking a specific group of muscle fibers with a high volume of work using a single exercise. The body adapts to this high amount of stress by hypertrophying the targeted muscle fibers.

For this method it is important to use "bigger bang for your buck" exercises. Barbell squats are better than leg extensions and barbell bench presses are better than dumbbell flies or pec-dec machines. In addition we implemented some accessory exercises to enhance the primary movements and to fill out the overall plan.

This was the block that we saw the greatest improvements by far. Not only did he nail the 20lb. gain by the end of this block, he was also doing multiple reps with his old 1 rep maximums in his primary indicator lifts. It is very common, when the proper loads are used and proper calories consumed, to make huge jumps in muscle mass and strength following this protocol.

THE TRAINING: IRON SHARPENS MAN

SAMPLE TRAINING WEEK FROM BLOCK 2

Monday, 11/18/13 - chest & back
1a. bench press: 95x10 / 10
1b. seated row: 70x10 / 10
2a. Incline dumbbell flye: 20x15 / 3
2b. Lat pulldown: 60x15 / 3

Wednesday, 11/20/13 - legs & abs
1. Trap bar dead lift: 155x3, 175x3, 200x3
2a. Squat: 125x10 / 10 sets
2b. Glute/hamstring raise: bwx10 / 10 sets
3a. Weighted sit-ups: 25x25 / 3 sets
3b. Calves: 40x15 / 3 sets

Friday, 11/22/13 - arms & shoulders
1a. Skull crusher: 40x10 / 10 sets
1b. Barbell curl: 45x10 / 10 sets
2a. Shrug: 95x12-15 / 3 sets
2b. Chest-supported rear lateral: 15x12-15 / 3 sets
2c. Laterals: 15x12-15 / 3 sets

TRAINING BLOCK 3 CUTTING PHASE

Duration: Current Plan

Objective: Maintain as much muscle and strength as possible while decreasing the extra body-fat that was gained during the first two training blocks.

In this training block the primary goal was to maintain as much of the new lean mass gained as possible, while reducing body-fat to improve muscle definition. This is typically referred to as a "cutting phase". Then, once optimal body-fat levels are achieved this becomes the maintenance plan until it is time to start detailing a plan for a future goal.

In this plan we also added some sprint work and interval training to his running, as well as adding some conditioning-based work in the gym such as high repetition kettle bell swings and weighted sled sprints.

SAMPLE TRAINING WEEK FROM BLOCK 3

Monday, 6/16/14
1. squat: barx10, 95x10, 135x8, 185x6, 225x4, 135x15
2a. Double kettle bell front squat: 16kgx10-12 / 3
2b. Glute/hamstring raise: 20x10-12 / 3
3a. Calves: 40x20-25 / 3
3b. 3-way abs: 25x25 / 3
3c. 2-arm kettle bell swings: 20kgx25/20/15/10/5
4. Sprints w/ weighted sled + 50lbs x 30yds / 10

Wednesday, 6/18/14
1. Bench press: barx15, 95x10, 115x8; 140x5, 155x3, 175x1
2. Incline dumbbell bench press: 35x15 / 3
3. Skull crushers: 45x15 / 3
4. Pushdowns: 50x15 / 2

THE TRAINING: IRON SHARPENS MAN

5. Lateral raise: 15x8-10 / 3
6. Rear deltoid raise: 15x8-10 / 2
7. Med ball abs: 10x25 / 4

Friday, 6/20/14

1. Trap bar dead lift: 135x5, 185x5; 225x5, 255x3, 285x1
2. Pull-ups: bw x 5/4/3/2/1 x 3 sets
3. Lat-pulldown: 100x12-15 / 3
4. Seated row: 100x10-12 / 2
5. Barbell curl: 60x10-12 / 3
6. Incline dumbbell curl: 20x12-15 / 2
7. Reverse sit-up/dragon flag: bwx25 / 4

PROGRESS TABLE

THIS TABLE WILL SHOW YOU THE INFORMATION ON STIC'S BODY COMPOSITION AND INDICATOR LIFTS THAT WE COLLECTED BEFORE, DURING, AND AFTER OUR PROJECT.

METRICS / DATES	PRE-GOAL ASSESSMENT 10/23/13	POST GOAL ASSESSMENT 1/13/14	CURRENT STATISTICS
Scale Weight	168 lbs.	188 lbs.	180 lbs.
Body Fat %	9.42%	10.36%	7.94%
Total Lean Mass	152.54 lbs.	168.53 lbs.	165.7 lbs.
Total Body Fat	15.86 lbs.	19.47 lbs.	14.3 lbs.
Squat	155x5; 205x1	205x4; 225x2	225x8; 275x1
Bench Press	115x5; 155x1	155x4; 175x2	135x25; 155x8; 170x6; 205x1
Trap Bar Dead lift	175x5; 245x1	245x3	275x3; 305x1

THE TRAINING: IRON SHARPENS MAN

You will notice that according to the table above his present scale weight is 8 lbs. lighter than his goal. The reason for this is when attempting to put on a significant amount of muscle mass, invariably a small amount of body-fat comes with it. Except in the case of a beginner who has never trained before, it is almost impossible to burn fat and gain muscle simultaneously.

Take competitive bodybuilders for instance, they are meticulous with their diet and training leading up to a competition and in the final cutting phase their goal is to maintain as much muscle as they can that was built in the off-season as they are stripping the fat off their body.

The 20 lb. gain led to Stic looking much thicker, but a little smoother than he liked. No problem, I told him in advance this would happen and that we would dedicate some time after the 20 lb. gain to reducing his body-fat percentage while maintaining as much of his new muscle mass as possible. To see the net changes look at his pre-goal assessment and his current stats and you will see that he is carrying 13 lbs. more lean mass and 1.5 lbs. less total body-fat now.

Those are great numbers when you factor that we burned off 5 lbs. of fat, the additional 4 he put on during the gaining phase and an extra pound-and-a-half on top of that, and only lost about 3 lbs. of the lean mass we put on during the gaining phase. It's important to keep in mind that when I use the term "lean mass" that represents everything in the body that is not fat. In addition to muscle it is water, blood, bone, etc..

The indicator lift improvement speaks for itself. He put 70 lbs. on his squat max and is able to do 8 repetitions with 20 lbs. more than his original 1 rep max. He put 50 lbs. on his bench press and is able to do 8 repetitions with his original 1 rep max. Finally, he put 60 lbs. on his trap-bar dead lift and is able to do 3 repetitions with 30 lbs. more than his original 1 rep max.

I've said, and seen, this before numerous times, if you want to get bigger, get stronger!

Two of the most dominant Mr. Olympia body-building champions, Dorian Yates and Ronnie Coleman (together they held the title for 14 years, Dorian for 6 and Ronnie for 8!) were known for using incredibly heavy weights in training. I've seen pictures of Dorian using over 400 lbs. in the barbell row and there are videos of Ronnie doing 800 lbs. for 2 in the squat and dead lift on YouTube. These two were not only two of the most dominant champions in the sport of bodybuilding, they both possessed very powerful and dense physiques, even when you compare them to the people at the top of the sport today.

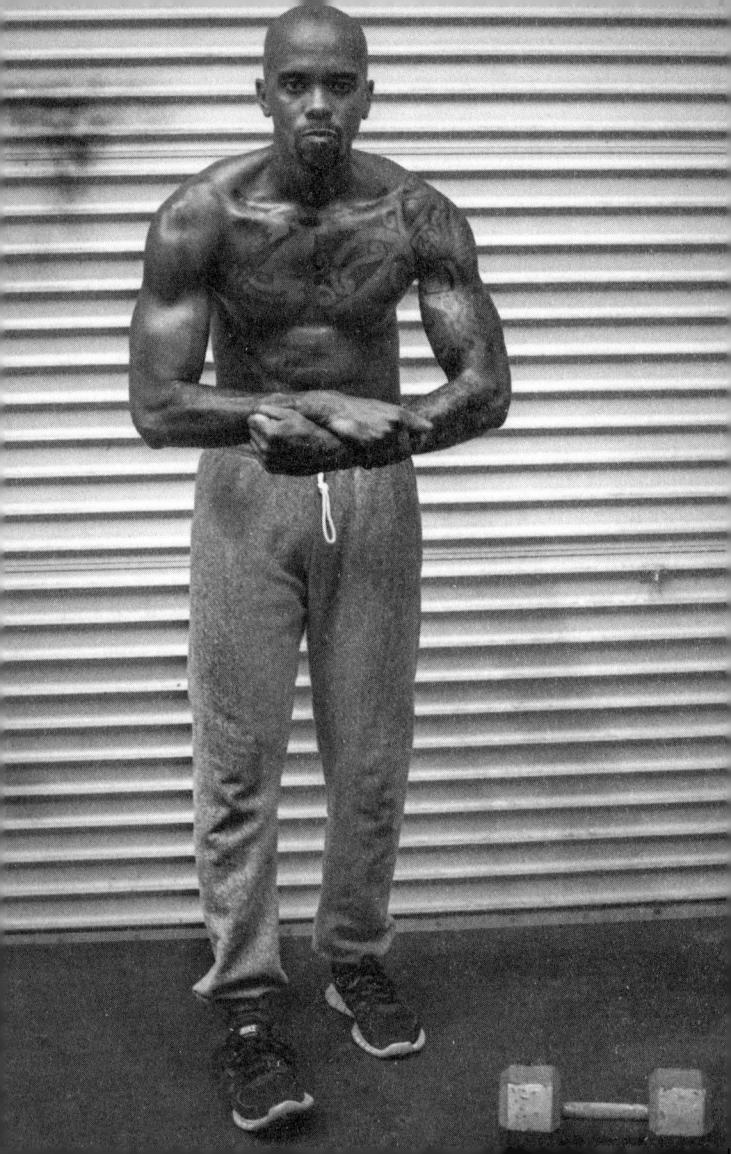

CHAPTER 20
FORM AND FOCUS

"I tell a student that the most important class you can take is technique. A great chef is first a great technician. 'If you are a jeweller, or a surgeon or a cook, you have to know the trade in your hand. You have to learn the process. You learn it through endless repetition until it belongs to you."
- JACQUES PEPIN

I cannot emphasize enough the importance of exercise technique. This is one of the reasons I purposely started Stic's program with a 3-4 week introductory block. We used this time to build excellent technique in the lifts that would make up the bulk of his training program.

When I work with clients in my training center, technique is always the limiting factor when it comes to adding weight to the bar. Proper technique minimizes the risk for injury when lifting heavy weights and it gives you the chance to progress more quickly.

It is far better to spend extra time when you start strength training practicing the lifts and building proper form and technique, then it is to do a movement incorrectly and have to correct bad form later.

THE TRAINING: IRON SHARPENS MAN

PROPER PRACTICE PREVENTS POOR PERFORMANCE

The more you do something, the more your brain and central nervous system engrain that pattern. It's like riding a bike. At first you can't balance the bicycle and you are wobbling all over the place. After a while not only can you balance on the bike, but you can ride without focusing on what you are doing, possibly to the point that you can ride with no hands, pop wheelies, or launch your bike off of BMX ramps. Once you reach that level, simply riding a bike requires no thought as you've ingrained that movement pattern into your nervous system.

Lifting weights is exactly like riding a bike. If you learn how to do a barbell squat incorrectly, and you practice this incorrect pattern over and over and over, your nervous system will program this poor technique. It will require far more work to fix it later on down the road than it does to spend a little extra time early on learning the squat pattern correctly. Once you have developed proficiency in the movement and it becomes ingrained in your nervous system you will be able to add weight and progress quickly, and most important safely, through the movement.

OUTSIDE FACTORS, DEALING WITH ADVERSITY, AND MISSING WORKOUTS.

At some point in your training things will not go your way. Real life happens and you may have to miss workouts or adjust your schedule. Learn to roll with these situations and don't allow them to get the best of you.

There will be times when you have a big workout planned and you get to the gym only to find that you are wiped out with nothing in the tank. Maybe your sleeping patterns were messed up, your nutrition has been bad, or maybe you've had to work crazy overtime at work and you are just plain tired. Going to the gym and expecting to hit personal records in all your lifts is not realistic at this point in time. No worries, just cut your training weights back a bit and reduce your overall training volume. Get a decent workout in, then get home, eat a healthy meal and get to bed early.

Having a training plan is very important, but know how to deviate from the plan when you need to.

THE UNIVERSITY OF ADVERSITY

Think about it like this, if you were driving from Atlanta to San Diego you would have a plan, a map or more likely in today's hi-tech world a navigation system of some sort. If the main route you were travelling was

THE TRAINING: IRON SHARPENS MAN

suddenly blocked due to an accident or construction, would you turn around and head home? Absolutely not. You would back-track, take a detour, or find an alternate route on your navigation system. Sure, it might add a little more time to your trip, but it will still keep you heading in the direction of your ultimate goal of reaching San Diego.

There are many other forms of adversity you may encounter other than just feeling a little tired at times. You may get sick, suffer an injury, or have to travel and not have access to a gym. Does this mean that you need to give up on your training? Absolutely not!

You get sick? Rest. Your body needs it. In addition to fighting off illness your muscles and nervous system will not be taxed and when you are well again it may lead to new gains and growth in your training.

You break your arm? No problem. Train the heck out of your legs, abs, and lower back. I did some training with a kettle bell fitness trainer a while back. He had been a competitive martial artist for many years. One of the things he is known for is his leg strength. He can do full range of motion one-legged squats, basically sit his butt on his calf while holding the other leg straight out in front of him. What makes this feat more impressive is that I've seen him do it while holding a pair of 88 lb. Kettle bells at his chest. He's not a very big guy either and that pair of 88 lb. kettle bells is pretty close to his body weight.

When I had asked him how he developed the ability to do this version of the one-legged squat so well, he explained that when he was training and competing with his full-contact martial arts team he had broken his arm. When the rest of his team was doing push-ups he began doing these one-legged squats and it took off from there. This just verifies that if you want to get really good at something make it a priority and put a lot of energy and focus into it.

WHERE THERE'S A WILL, THERE IS A WAY

You have to travel and this prevents you from getting to the gym? No problem, just do what you can. You can always to body weight squats, push-ups, lunges, and various abdominal exercises in your hotel room with no equipment. Get creative. Shortly after Stic hit his goal of a 20 lb. gain he had to go on tour in Europe, something like 18 shows in 21 days. He had every intention of hitting the gym but it never happened. What did he do? He did body weight squats, push-ups and abs in his hotel room. He loaded up his suitcase and used it for triceps extensions, curls, and 1-arm rows. Simply put, he made due.

While it wasn't the same as getting to the gym and hoisting the iron, it was certainly better than nothing and it made all the difference when he got back to my

THE TRAINING: IRON SHARPENS MAN

training center. Had he said "screw it" and blown off those 3 weeks he would have lost much of his progress and we would have had to work even harder to get him back on track.

Remember, overcoming resistance is not just about pushing a barbell off your chest. It is about taking those lessons you learn in the gym on the lifting platform and applying them to the situations you encounter in your life. Do not strive to build an iron body only; build an iron mind as well.

CHAPTER 21
THE BIG SIX: KEY EXERCISES FOR STRENGTH AND MASS

*"Knowing is not enough, we must apply.
Willing is not enough, we must do."*
- BRUCE LEE

I am often asked what the best exercises for strength and muscle mass gain are, and without a doubt they are the 5 big, basic, compound (i.e. Multiple joints) barbell lifts plus pull-ups. Six exercises, that's all! I know that after I present this list you might wonder where the curls and crunches are. I'm not saying isolation exercises like dumbbell curls or lateral raises are not important, they definitely have their place. What is most important is building the foundation, and nothing leads to great strength and mass increases than this short list of compound exercises performed with progressively heavier weights.

Without further adieu, here are the best exercises that you can do to add slabs of muscle to your physique and improve your strength levels almost immediately. The are the primary exercises that should make up the core of your program. These should never be replaced by smaller isolation exercises. I'm not saying that doing barbell or dumbbell curls is bad, they are a great exercise for the biceps, but doing pull-ups and

THE TRAINING: IRON SHARPENS MAN

rows will build the biceps while hitting the lats and upper back muscles. Please note that this list is in no particular order.

- Barbell squat
- Barbell dead lift
- Barbell bench press
- Barbell row
- Standing overhead barbell press
- Pull-up

If you are looking for some accessory exercises to supplement the primary movement I'd recommend the following.

- Good morning
- Romanian dead lift
- Step up
- Split squat or 1-leg squat
- 1-arm dumbbell row
- Inverted row
- Shrug
- Rear-delt raise
- Bench press with dumbbells
- Shoulder press with dumbbells
- Push-ups
- Dips barbell curls
- Dumbbell curls
- Barbell triceps extension
- Dumbbell triceps extension

- Sit-ups
- Reverse sit-ups

If you would like instructions for these exercises and to see them performed correctly, visit my YouTube page at www.youtube.com/user/sshetler13 and go to the playlist section. There you will find play lists divided by categories such as upper body pushing exercises, upper body pulling exercises, etc.. This is a free resource that I wanted to make available online so that anyone could have access to solid performance tips for basic strength training exercises.

HEAVY WEIGHTS AND LOW REPS VS. LIGHT WEIGHTS AND HIGHER REPS

Which is better? First I would say, why limit yourself. In order to fully develop muscle mass both protocols have their place. That being said, I think that training with heavy weights is often overlooked when building muscle is the goal.

Granted, high volume training with moderately heavy weights produces fantastic gains in muscle mass, as you saw in the second block of Stic's training plan, but at some point you have to get stronger. If Stic repeated that exact same cycle a second time he would not get the same benefit. See your body adapts to exercise. It adapts to the amount of weight used on strength exercises, it adapts to the speed that you run at, and

THE TRAINING: IRON SHARPENS MAN

so one and so forth. This is how we progress, we push the body and it adapts to that stimulus. Then we push a little harder and it adapts again.

Lifting heavy weights, I would define heavy as using a 1-5 rep max load, some of the time is essential. As you raise your maximal strength levels, you will be able to perform your volume work with heavier weights which will ultimately lead to great gains in both strength and muscle mass.

Consider this example. Let's say that your 1-rep max in the bench press is 225 and you just finished a 6-week high volume cycle of the 10x10 program Stic used. You started with 135 (60% of 225) for 10x10 on the bench press. Following this volume cycle you focused on improving your maximal strength and raised your bench press up to 250 for a new 1-rep max. If you were to do another 10x10 cycle, your starting weight would now be 150 (60% of 250) for the 10 sets of 10. This would create a much higher volume and your body would respond much better than it would if you repeated the cycle with the weight you used before.

How much different? Consider the total volume. When using 135 for 10 sets of 10 your total volume is 13,500 lbs. When using 150 for 10 sets of 10 your total volume is 15,000 lbs. A full 1,500 lbs. more total volume than your first cycle and a much greater stress for your body to adapt to.

By raising your maximal strength levels you were able to expose your body to a higher stimulus on your next volume cycle. This is why it is essential that you keep a training log and track your workouts. If you are not steadily adding more weight to your lifts, your gains will come to a halt very quickly.

Keep in mind, I'm not suggesting that you need to be a power lifter, but training with maximal, or near-maximal weights some of the time will add strength quickly and help you build dense muscle mass fast.

STRENGTH TRAINING WHILE GETTING RIPPED

Now that we've established that it is essential to lift heavy weights to get strong and build muscle, what about when it's time to strip off the body fat to display all the newly acquired muscle mass?

I know there is a popular myth that the best way to get ripped is to lift with lighter weights and higher reps. Trust me, that is just a myth. If you stop training with heavy weights you will not maintain the strength and muscle you built during the gaining phase.

Granted, you will most likely see a slight drop in your strength when you begin cutting. This is usually due to two reasons.

First, when your goal is burning fat, this generally requires a reduction in calories. Even Stic, who is

THE TRAINING: IRON SHARPENS MAN

naturally lean and skinny had to manipulate his diet in order to cut the fat. Second, a cutting phase usually incorporates greater amounts of cardio. I know many bodybuilders who do very little to no cardio when they are in a gaining phase, but during a cutting phase may do up to 2 hours a day.

When you are expending that much energy, and eating less food, you will lose some strength. However you should still train as heavy as possible to prevent losing muscle mass during a cutting phase.

Do not worry about how much strength you lose when you are cutting, unless you are going to extremes and preparing for a bodybuilding contest it won't be much.

CHAPTER 22
BUILDING IN BALANCE

"Man who chases two rabbits catches neither."
- CONFUCIUS

It is very difficult, next to impossible, to gain large amounts of muscle mass and strength while simultaneously cutting body fat. It is something that beginner trainees may be able to do, but there will come a point in time that you'll need to choose a goal and focus on it 100% if you are serious about your progress.

If you do not have any short term goals, and are happy with your body fat level, the appropriate course of action would be to focus on adding strength and muscle mass slowly over a period of years. This may not be the case for many. Some of you may want to get big fast. The drawback to putting mass on fast is that you will have to be willing to put on some body fat.

This was the boat Stic was in. His goal of 20 lbs. in 4 months was pretty big for such a short time frame. That's OK, I was up-front with him and told him that he'd have to be willing to put on a little body fat and smooth out a bit, but we could take that off later.

THE TRAINING: IRON SHARPENS MAN

Before we even began training we set what we agreed would be acceptable limits for extra body-fat gain. Since he was starting off at 9% I suggested that allowing himself to go up to 11 or 12% would be fine, and pretty easy to take off after the 20lb. gain. It ended up we didn't even need a 2-3% body fat cushion. At the 20lb. mark his body fat had only increased by 0.9%!

This just reiterates my statement about not being able to serve two masters simultaneously. Even with a high metabolism and being naturally skinny, coupled with the fact he was still doing a decent amount of cardio, Stic still put on body fat. Not much, but enough to smooth him out and get him worried. Let's just say he wasn't a big fan of the little Buddha-belly he had going on!

The beauty of gaining all that extra muscle is this; the more muscle mass you carry, the more calories you burn, even at rest. Why? Muscle is more metabolically active than fat. It requires more calories to sustain itself at work and at rest. So even if you are just sitting there doing nothing, your muscle is burning more calories to sustain itself than your fat is.

Due to this the cutting phase was pretty easy. He had about 16 lbs. of new muscle working for him that not only improved his training metabolism, but his resting metabolism as well. Simply put, more muscle means more calories burned.

Here is my advice when trying to decide what to do. If you are naturally lean, I'd consider this to be 8-9% body fat or under with somewhat visible abs, go ahead and focus on gaining muscle. If you are carrying around too much body fat, focus on cleaning up the diet and getting lean. Chances are if you are not training and you are carrying around excessive body-fat, you will build muscle regardless, at least for the first few months of your initial program.

Many people like to use the winter months as their gaining months for a couple of reasons. First, the winter months contain some of the bigger holidays, and with the festivities comes eating, and usually a lot of it. Don't use your gaining phase as an excuse to eat a bunch of crap, but this would be the time to not sweat a cheat meal here or there. Also, unless you live in tropical regions, the winter months are usually cold and this means long pants and sleeves and less showing off the body.

After a few months of gaining strength and mass people will generally focus their efforts on burning body-fat through the spring time, so that when summer hits they are ripped and ready to hang out at the pool or beach.

This is exactly what Stic did. We focused on gaining mass from November through January, then when he got back from his tour at the end of February we went

THE TRAINING: IRON SHARPENS MAN

right into the cutting and maintenance phase.

We decided the maintenance phase would allow him to maintain a level of muscle mass and body-fat that he was happy with while still be able to excel at his health and fitness goals. For Stic this represented a net gain of about 13 lbs. of lean mass and a reduction of almost 2% body fat. So now he's considerably heavier and walking around at 7% body fat! This is solid proof that goal setting couple with hard work and attention to detail will get you where you want to be every time.

THREE ELEMENTS OF VIBRANT HEALTH

Here are a few key points that I feel were imperative to Stic's success that you can take from this project if you aspire to build strength and mass quickly.

First, you must provide the body with the nutrients it needs. This is as simple as eating a 100% whole food, plant-based diet, and drinking fresh, clean water. You don't need supplements, powders, pills, energy drinks, or drugs.

Second, you must strengthen the mind and spirit. Adopt an energy cultivation practice such as yoga, qigong, Tai Chi, and / or meditation. Get control of your mind and energize your body. In addition, get plenty of rest and learn to relax.

Third, you must strengthen the body. Lift weights and provide the stimulus necessary for the body to get stronger. Challenge the cardiovascular system to get stronger by running, swimming, biking, or something similar. Stretch your muscles and mobilize your joints, because if you don't use them you will lose them.

TIPS FOR MUSCLE BUILDING SUCCESS

Here are a few key points that I feel were imperative to Stic's success that you can take from this project if you aspire to build strength and mass quickly.

1. SET A GOAL.

This is crucial. Always have a goal for your training. This allows you to stay on track and stay focused on your training. It will also prevent you from program hopping. Jumping from program to program is a surefire way to halt progress. Setting a goal will make each and every training session you do to get there meaningful. Each training session builds on the other until gradually you get closer and closer to your goal. Without a goal it's very easy to skip training sessions or just "go through the motions" when you are in the gym.

Don't make your goal too easy or too hard. If it is too easy you will not get anything out of the process of achieving it. If it is too hard you may very well become

THE TRAINING: IRON SHARPENS MAN

discouraged and give up when you get there. While 1,000 lb. squats are possible, and more and more power lifters cross that barrier every year, setting that as a goal when your squat is only 200 lbs. may not be a good idea. Get to 300 lbs. first!

Set a goal that challenges you and makes you a little uncomfortable, but make sure it is within reach. It could also be part of a bigger goal. Maybe your ultimate goal is to go from a 200 lb. to a 300 lb. squat in a year. Your 6-month goal could be a 250 lb. squat and your 3-month goal could be a 225 lb. squat. By breaking a large goal up into smaller goals you are creating the opportunity for smaller successes more frequently and by hitting each small goal you are closer and closer to your big goal.

2. SET A DEADLINE.

Set a deadline for your goal. Giving yourself a deadline puts pressure on you to accomplish your goal. It will keep your attention focused on that goal and give you more motivation to get everything out of your training that you can.

I always made my best progress in power lifting when I registered for a power lifting meet. Once I filled out the application and sent in the check I was committed! I was much more focused in each training session as after each session I was closer and closer to the competition. This was a great way to put positive pressure on myself and I always made my best gains in the months leading up to a meet.

3. EAT.

This should go without saying, but you have to eat! Eat to fuel your workouts and nourish your body. Consume the correct proteins, amino acids, carbohydrates, fats, vitamins, minerals, and enzymes. Get these nutrients from a healthy, whole food, and preferably plant-based diet. Not only will this have a very positive effect on your body, but it will have a positive effect on the environment and all sentient beings. Make sure your nutrition supports your goal. If you are eating clean 95% of the time, take that other 5% and enjoy your life. Just don't use it as an excuse to binge!

4. TRAIN.

I shouldn't have to spend a lot of time on this one. Training is essential. Training stimulates your body to adapt to stress and grow. Notice I said stimulate. Lately annihilation seems to be the goal for a lot of people. There is no reason to destroy yourself in the gym. Hit the body hard, hard enough to create the stimulus needed to grow, then get into rest and recovery mode. Get the healthy nutrients in your system so that you can get ready to train again.

THE TRAINING: IRON SHARPENS MAN

5. REST.

This is where the growth happens. Training breaks down your body, rest, recovery, and nutrition is where the body adapts and grows. The healthy food you eat brings essential nutrients to the muscles allowing them to rebuild and grow. The rest encourages this growth. If you are training every day and not allowing your body to recover, you will eventually stall in your progress and most likely regress. Growth happens outside of the gym, provided you did the necessary work in the gym.

6. STAY MOTIVATED.

Don't lose sight of your goal. If you set the goal then the goal is worthy of your time. Stay on track and never quit. Training can be a metaphor for life. When it gets challenging and you feel like giving up, that is when you need to grit down and do it the most. Training is challenging, just as life is challenging at times.

Challenges present opportunity for growth. When you challenge your muscles by slapping another 45lb. plate on each side of the barbell, you are giving your body an opportunity to grow and become stronger. When challenges happen in your life, they are usually opportunities for you to grow and become stronger. There are a lot of lessons in that rusty pile of iron, all you have to do is watch and listen for them.

7. FOCUS ON THE PROGRESS.

Having a goal and deadline is critical to your success, but don't be married to it! It's important to learn to enjoy the journey. The progress is where the real fun happens, where the lessons are learned, and where the personal growth occurs. I always have a goal for my training, whether or not I hit it by my deadline does not matter. I can always push the deadline back. The goal for me serves to keep my training on track and prevents me from getting distracted.

Power lifting meets and kettle bell sport competitions are fun. They give me the opportunity to test myself. The camaraderie at these events is awesome, and it's always great to get together and compete with your friends and other like-minded individuals. However the training is what I really love!

I love walking into my private gym where it is just the iron and me. It's part of my daily ritual. It's my zen. It's a meditative experience. When I am lifting all my focus is in the present moment. It's not on the project I need to get done for next week, the book I'm currently writing, the clients I have coming in, or the guy who cut me off in traffic that morning. My focus is 100% in the moment, the here and now, this iron that I am lifting. Every fiber of my being is engaged in that present moment. I love the progress, and I encourage you to love it too.

THE TRAINING: IRON SHARPENS MAN

8. IF YOU GET OFF TRACK, DON'T STRESS OUT, SIMPLY GET BACK ON TRACK.

If you are driving down the road and you get a flat tire, do you get out and slash the other three tires? No. You fix the flat and move on. Now what if you get off your nutrition plan? Do you use that as an excuse to binge and say, "screw it, I blew it so I might as well go big." Unfortunately this happens a lot. Guess what, there will be times where you get off track. We all do. No worries, just get back on track.

If you blow your nutrition for one meal, enjoy it! Call it a reward meal for sticking to a healthy plan the majority of the time, then just get back on to healthy eating. The same goes for training, if you miss a workout don't sweat it. Just get back in the gym the next day! Or do what Stic did and just improvise. When he was on a short tour in Europe he had to perform daily, this prevented him from getting out and finding a gym to train in. He made due. He did some calisthenics and used his luggage as weights and did what he could in the hotel room. Is it ideal? No. Is it better than nothing and shows how committed he was to accomplishing his goal? Absolutely!

9. COMMIT TO YOUR GOAL 100%.

If you set a goal and decide that it is worth your time be sure to follow it through. If it is worth giving time out of your life to then commit to it. Commit to it with enthusiasm, passion, and love. Put your heart and soul into it so that you will inspire others with your ambition and drive. I heard someone say once, "Don't ask yourself if you are worthy of your goals, instead ask are your goals worthy of you?"

10. DO NOT SACRIFICE YOUR HEALTH TO GET BIGGER AND STRONGER.

My friend and colleague, Dr. Lou Pack, once said, "Health is something we go through on the way to fitness." I couldn't agree more. Look at any of the popular muscle magazines on the newsstand. Up to 30%, or more of the pages are ads for supplements that are supposed to burn fat or build muscle.

The things people do to become what we perceive of as "fit" are often far from healthy. People go to extremes to look fit, and often sacrifice their health in the process. I've found that if you focus on becoming healthy on the inside, the outside will always reflect it. It is possible to get strong, build muscle, get lean, and improve athletic performance without sacrificing your health.

Push your body to the limit, see what it is capable of, but treat it well. It is your soul's temple, and if you take care of it as such you will experience health and vitality all the way up until your final days. Do not resign

THE TRAINING: IRON SHARPENS MAN

yourself to the fact that we degenerate and become sick and unwell with age. Be healthy, be vibrant, and kick ass until it is time to move on to the next stage of being!

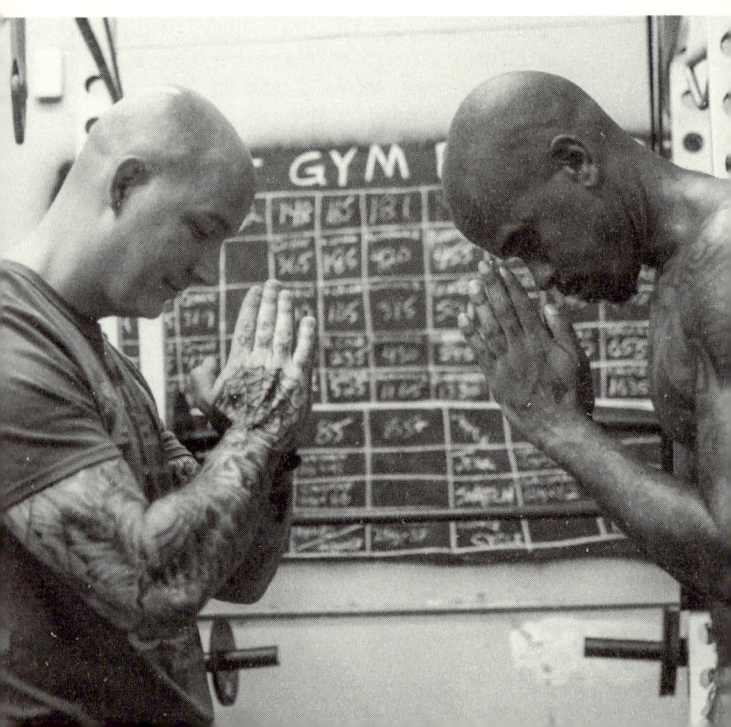

CHAPTER 23
PHYSICAL CULTURE:
WHY WE NEED TO GET BACK TO IT

"The knowledge of one's strength entails a real mastery over oneself; it breeds energy and courage, helps one over the most difficult tasks of life, and procures contentment and true enjoyment of living."
- GEORGE HACKENSCHMIDT

Around the late 1800's and early 1900's those who trained for strength were referred to as physical culturists. The concept of physical culture is what we think of today as physical fitness or "gym life".

Back then, those who trained focused on total human development, a strong mind and body. They trained to possess great strength, a lean and muscular physique, vibrant health, and a strong mind. They ate well, the trained appropriately, they knew how to relax, and were well educated.

In contrast, today most people are specialists. They train for ultra endurance, bodybuilding, weight lifting, etc.. Please understand I am not condemning athletes, I understand that if you are going to compete at the highest levels in sport, specialization rules. Unfortunately, to be a high level athlete today, it often comes at the expense of your health. That doesn't

THE TRAINING: IRON SHARPENS MAN

mean that an athlete shouldn't be as healthy as possible, and look to regain their health when their competitive days are through. If you choose to pursue professional, or high level athletics that is a sacrifice you might have to make.

That being said, I think the notion of physical culture applies to the vast majority of the population to who want to be lean, strong, healthy, and vibrant. This cannot be accomplished by lifting weights alone. In order to possess truly abundant health we must develop our mind, body, and spirit. To do this effectively reinventing the wheel is completely unnecessary. All we need to do is look back 100+ years ago to what the founding fathers of physical culture did. Men like Arthur Saxon, George Hackenschmidt, and Eugene Sandow.

Side note, the trophy awarded to the winner of the Mr. Olympia contest is actually a statue of Mr. Sandow and is simply referred to as "The Sandow". Sandow possessed what many consider to be the ideal physique which is why his statue is used as the top award for the highest level of bodybuilding competition, although today there is a bit of contradiction with this notion.

George "The Russian Lion" Hackenschmidt said, "Health can never be divorced from strength." Wise words from a physical culture legend.

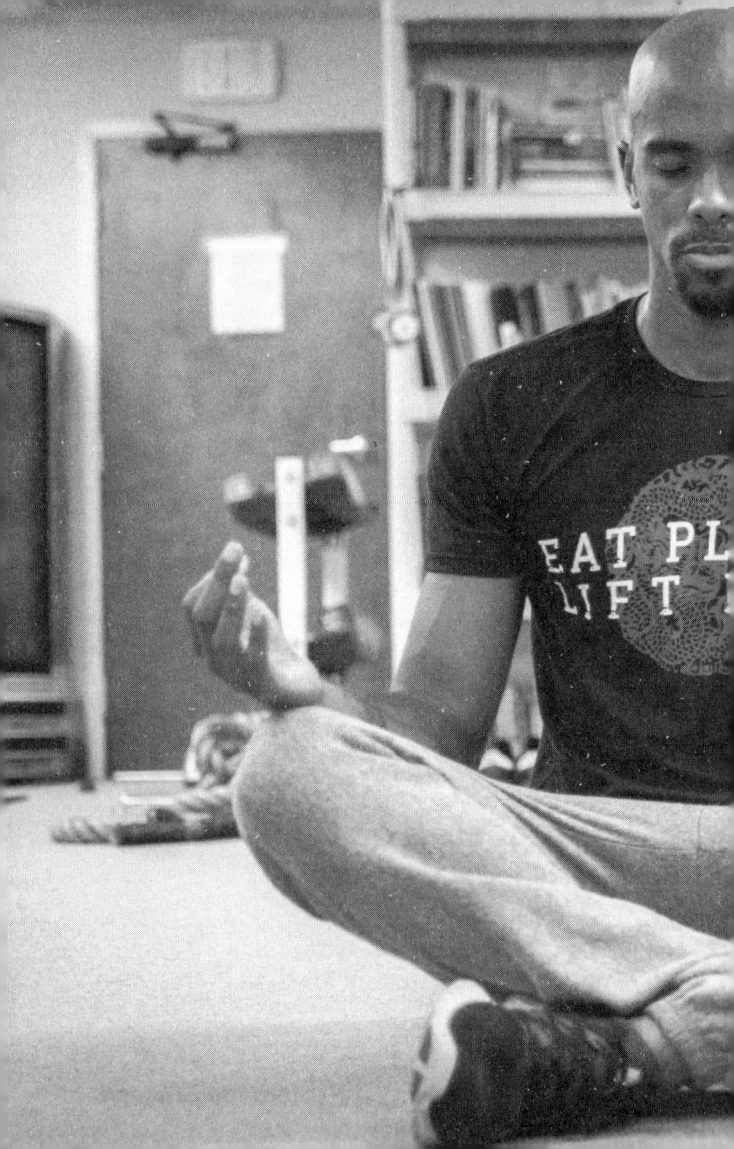

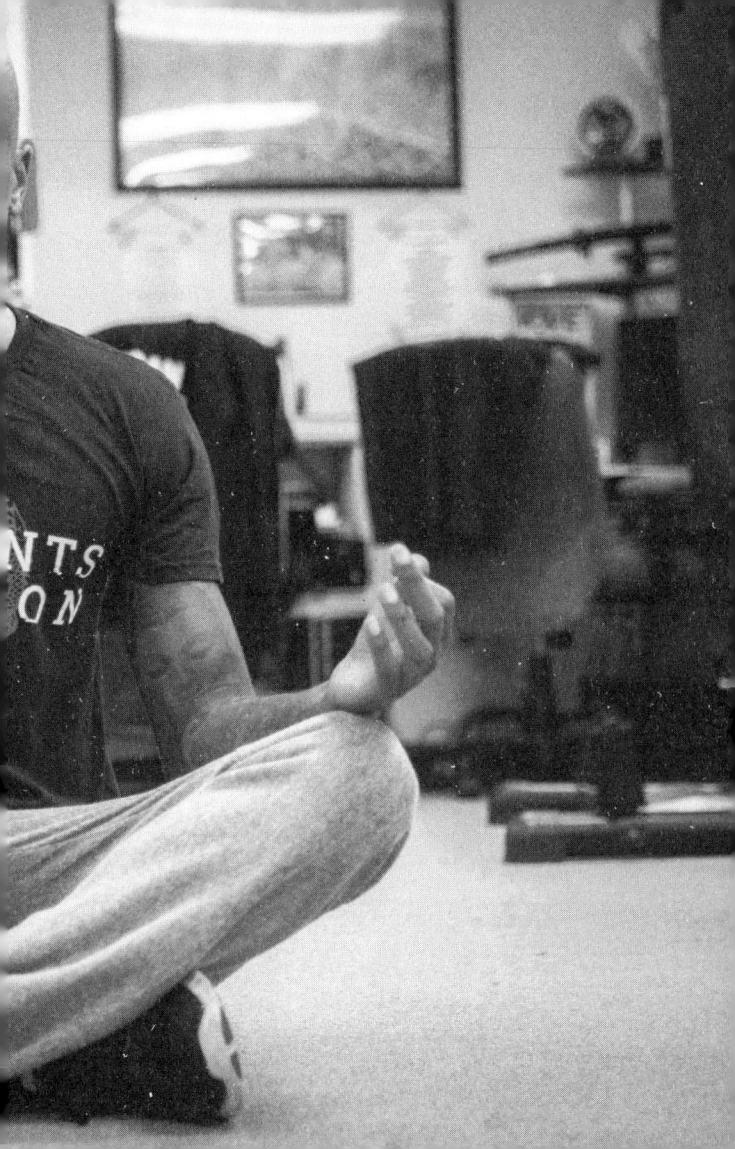

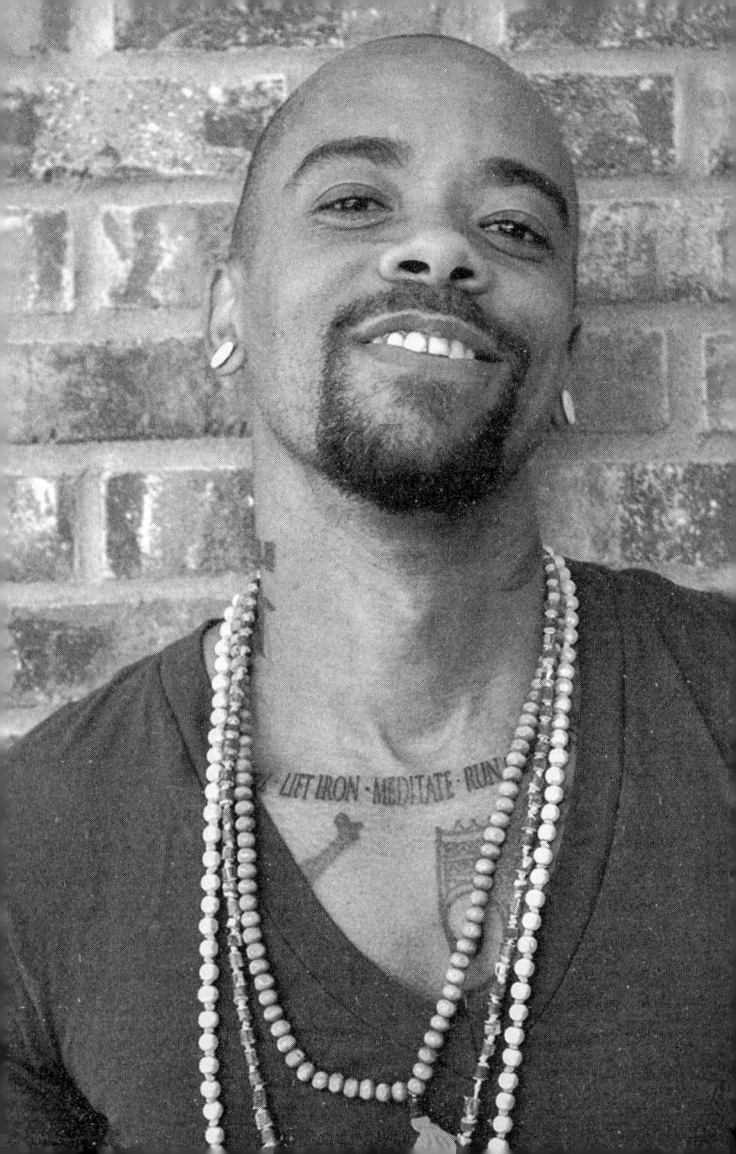

KHNUM "STIC" IBOMU

Khnum "STIC" Ibomu is an internationally acclaimed Hip Hop artist, producer and writer as well as a passionate holistic health and fitness advocate. Stic created the ground breaking "fit hop" album "The Workout" that debuted at #1 of iTunes Fitness charts. Stic is the founder of the RBG FIT CLUB- a lifestyle brand movement and website fusing Hip hop Culture with holistic wellness. Stic has received the Black Men's Holistic Health Award and The Betty Shabazz Award for Social Justice. Stic meditates daily, loves long distance running, hot yoga and has practiced martial arts for over 10 years.

He lives in Atlanta with his son and his wife of over 21 years Holistic Nutritionist and Author Afya Ibomu.

Stic can be contacted for Workshops, Speaking Events, Live Performances and so on at Stic@rbgfitclub.com.

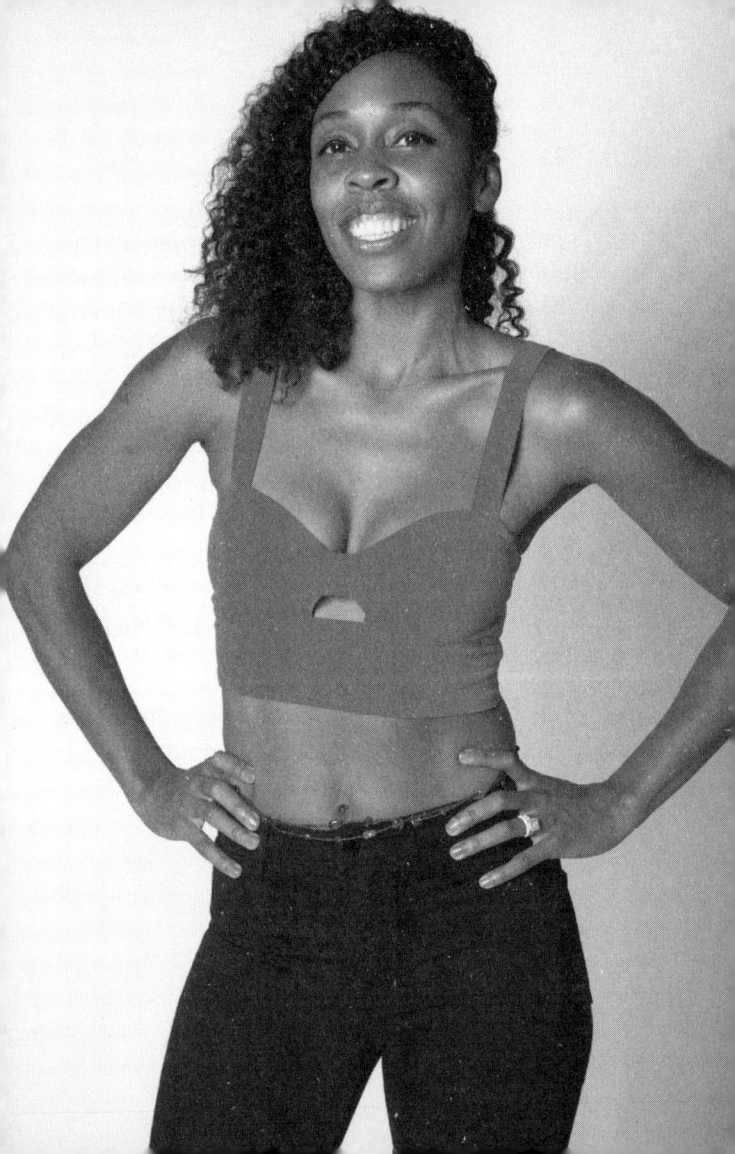

AFYA IBOMU

Afya Ibomu is a Holistic Nutritionist, the CEO of NATTRAL.com, and has been plant based since 1990. Her third book The Vegan Soul Food Guide to the Galaxy, was nominated for an African American Literary Award for cookbook of the year. Afya is certified in Holistic Health and holds a bachelor's degree in nutrition. She is also the author of the Get Your Crochet On! pattern book series, that have sold over 25,000 copies. Afya is a celebrity nutritionist and crochet designer working with hip hop artists such as Erykah Badu, Common, Dead Prez and Talib Kweli.

Afya currently conducts cooking demos and classes, teaches nutrition workshops and counsels fitness competitors. She lives in Atlanta with her husband stic of dead prez and their son Itwela.

Check out her allergy friendly, plant based cookbook The Vegan Remix and to keep up with what afya is doing, check her out on all social media platforms @afyaibomu

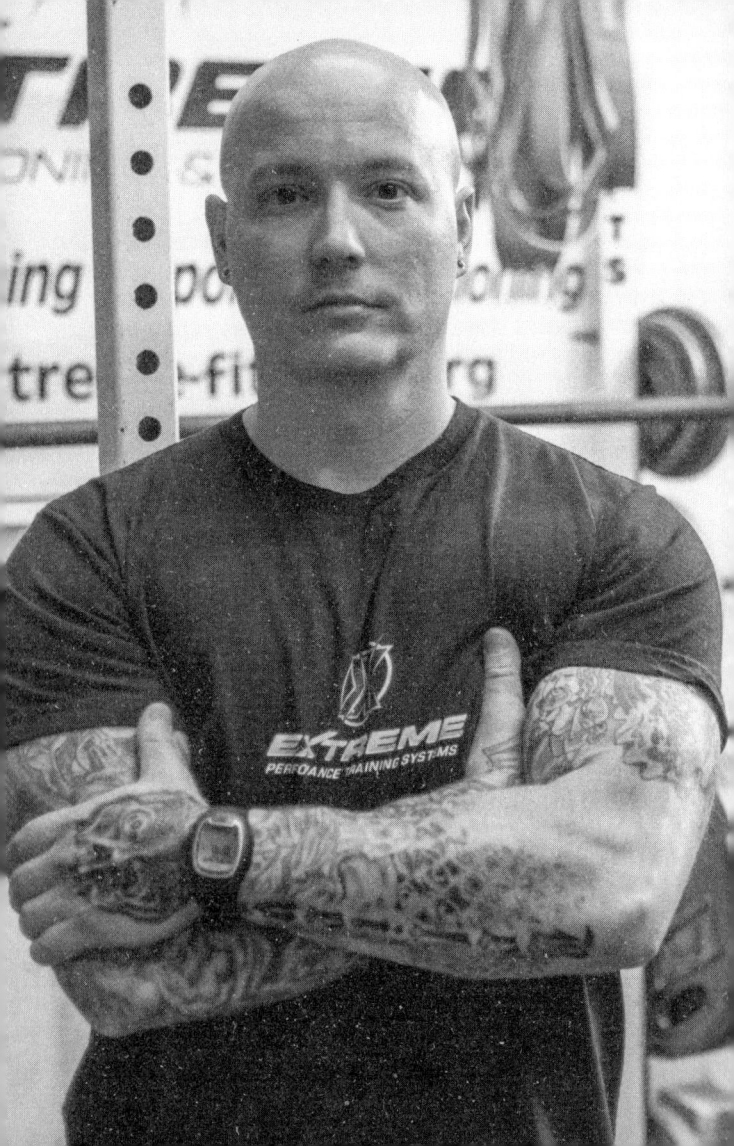

SCOTT SHETLER, NSCA-CPT

Scott is a holistic fitness professional with over 16 years of experience in the strength training, health, and fitness industry. He is the owner of the Atlanta-based private training center, Extreme Performance Training Systems; has a degree in Health and Physical Education; and is a certified personal trainer through the National Strength and Conditioning Association (NSCA).

He has authored 5 books and coauthored 3 books, on various topics related to strength training, health and fitness. In addition he consults with people worldwide through his online training and consulting business, and presents regularly at seminars and clinics.

Scott has competed in the strength sports of power lifting and kettle bell sport, is a member of Team Plantbuilt's power lifting team, and is a student of qigong and the internal martial art of Taijiquan. He believes in a holistic approach to human development, one that integrates the mind, body, and spirit equally.

Throughout his career he has trained numerous athletes from sports such as football, baseball, basketball, swimming, volleyball, tennis, parkour (free running), triathlon, jiu jitsu, mixed martial arts, bodybuilding, kettle bell sport, and power lifting, from recreational to professional levels. In addition he has helped many people lose weight, build muscle, and improve their health and quality of life.

Scott offers a variety of services both in-person and through the internet. To find out how he can help you with your personal health and fitness program visit him online at the following websites:

If you would like to work with him in person, or check out one of his books, visit www.extreme-fitness.org or his personal site www.scottshetler.com.

If you would like to consult with him online, visit www.onlinepersonaltrainerinfo.org.

If you would like to train live with him through his online fitness studio, visit www.powhow.com/classes/scott-shetlers-fitness-studio.

If you would like to help him support animal welfare, visit www.plantbasedperformance.org.

For Scott's most recent updates, follow him on these social media sites:

facebook.com/sshetlerfitness
facebook.com/ecfitness
twitter.com/sshetler